Dian Zhen Liao Fa

TCM and Electroherbalism

Esther E Aldrich

Randall R Bornemann

PUBLICATION NOTE:

Once again, we have decided to self-publish. As with our previous book, **Fang Xiang Liao Fa: Essential Oil Analogues of TCM Herbal Formulas**, we wanted to keep the price low for our readers. As always, we hope that, while the book might not be the fanciest volume on your shelf, the substantiveness of the content will make up for the plainness of its appearance.

REQUEST FOR FEEDBACK

We consider this to be a "beta" edition of this book. As self-publishing authors, we do not have access to professional copy editors. If you find errata, please notify us. Further, if you have ideas, suggestions or requests, also feel free to contact us. This book does not belong to us as authors. It belongs to the greater community of TCM practitioners and their patients.

tcmrandall@yahoo.com

Esther's Forward

I was first introduced to a frequency generator when I met my former NP and mentor **Paul Klebs**. He was a very unconventional person, but tirelessly devoted to organic foods, sustainable agriculture and sustainable herbs/medicine. If I needed food he fed me, if I needed water he gave me access to his well. And when I couldn't afford something he just gave it to me including enhancing my personal library with several books. He wasn't without his faults, but his compassion and generosity were what inspired me. Because so many herbs are not harvested sustainably, because so many natural resources are depleted, using frequencies became an area of interest for him. This interest he passed on to me.

Randall, my co-author, was the first person to introduce me to the works of **Nenah Sylver** and a video of paramecia exploding under the microscope when exposed to their Mortal Oscillatory Rate (MOR). **Dr. Chi**, one of my great instructors at AAAOM, then taught us specific frequencies to use while doing e-stim on patients in the clinic, based on Chinese research while **Randall** and I were getting our Masters Degrees in Chinese Medicine.

People who know me know that I like to take things to the next level of creativity. So, while I was doing my internship, **Randall** lent me a Rife machine, and I used it in place of the e-stim machines in the student clinic. The Rife had a broader frequency range, and I was curious.

Whenever I seem to have a wild idea people who are interested in wild ideas find me. One such person was a friend who has Lyme Disease. Then she referred another person and another. Our good friend and mentor **Soke W. Kent Bergstrom** had also been having people with Lyme coming to him in droves.

As someone who doesn't treat Western Diagnoses, I often found online frequency guides to be difficult. It became kind of a trial and error guessing game of which frequencies would match up with their TCM (Traditional Chinese Medicine) patterns, because everything was cataloged according to Allopathic Medicine.

At some point, I think the idea for the book culminated around our research project for a class, and **Randall,** always being one to dump gasoline and lit matches on my blazing ideas, quickly talked me into the project that has become this book.

Being a person who suffered from a lot of hypersensitivities and allergies I frequently attracted this type of patient and being a person who was eager to work with complementary care I was all too familiar with doctors not being comfortable with Chinese herbs, essential oils and really anything other than needles and electrical stimulation. Rife was something that I didn't have to worry as much about depleting natural resources, an allergic response or a doctor who was not in favor of our patient being on herbs. This was just an extension, an evolution of e-stim. It was safe, it was easy, and if my patients hated needles I could always apply the frequencies through the foot pads.

That, in a nut shell, is why we decided to put this book together. I want to dedicate this book to two people. The first is **Dr. Paul Klebs** for introducing me to Rife, the second is **Dr. Brian E. Briggs** (RIP) who introduced me to CAM (Complimentary Alternative Medicine). Without these guys I'd be teaching linguistics somewhere if I hadn't died from Thyroid Disease. I am eternally in your debt.

And to all my friends, family, teachers, mentors and colleagues who have always encouraged my unconventional self, a bridge is built with many stones, a tree is grown with many leaves, a fire is fed with much kindling. If I ever stand on another shore, if I ever grow in a barren place, if I ever burn brightly, it's because of all of you.

Esther Aldrich
Summer, 2013

Randall's Forward

We hope you all enjoy this book. We did not have the space to get too deeply into areas like pleomorphism. As with our previous book, we wanted to make sure we kept the price down so that the book would be accessible to our readers.

Therefore we've glossed over quite a bit of material that we would otherwise have covered more in depth. This includes biographical material about both **Royal Raymond Rife** and **George Lakhovsky**.

Our main goal is to show the basics of "how to do it." If we have accomplished that, we will consider ourselves successful. There is far more information included in other volumes, such as **Nenah Silver**'s excellent **Handbook of Rife Frequency Therapy** if people are interested. We can't recommend **Nenah**'s book strongly enough. We also plan on researching the similarities and compatibilities between pleomorphism and the TCM paradigm of pathogenesis in a future volume.

I would like to give special thanks to our good friend and mentor **Soke W. Kent Bergstrom.** With all his years of experience and lore, **Kent**'s wisdom and general insights continue to be invaluable. From his training with the legendary **Robert** and **Tina Sohn**, to his decades of experience in martial arts to his personal wisdom and years of experience in healing, **Kent** embodies for us, what this field is all about.

In addition to **Kent** and **Nenah**, I also dedicate this book to **Dr. Mengnai Li**, an exceptional surgeon, who performed miracles on my joints, but who doesn't know how to kill MRSA.

Finally, I would like to thank my co-author **Esther Aldrich** for all her help, ingenuity and frankly, hard work and devotion to this project. **Esther** did the original presentation in **Dr. Liu's** class on Science and Acupuncture. She spoke for an hour and a half, showed some videos and had people spellbound.

Thank you so much **Esther**, for all the hours in the clinic and classrooms. You really ran with the idea of converting electroherbalism into TCM, and none of this would have been possible without your enthusiasm and self discipline.
Randall Bornemann
Summer 2013

Epistemological Note

Here are our major objections to "Science," or more specifically "The Scientific Method" as a rigorous epistemology:

1: Scientific knowledge is not possible.
As **Karl R. Popper** demonstrates in **The Logic of Scientific Discovery**, the empirical method only *DIS*proves previous theories and hypotheses. Positive knowledge is beyond its purview.

2: The Empirical Method is based on numerous superstitions that have been discredited for the past 2-3 centuries.
"Science" is based on many superstitions, such as objecthood, identity across time, efficient causality, third person reality, the idea that the universe operates according to "laws," the idea that these laws are objectively knowable, etc. See also **Enquiry Concerning Human Understanding** by **David Hume**, **Philosophical Writings** of **Charles Sanders Peirce** and **Process and Reality and Science and the Modern World** by **Alfred North Whitehead**.

3: The reasoning of science is based on inductive reasoning, which is NOT logically valid.
Inductive reasoning consists of reasoning from the particular to the general. For example, we can observe 1001 white swans. From this we conclude that all swans are white. However, this is only a theory, and it only takes one black swan to disprove this theory.

4: "Science" has been separated from religion.
Western empirical science excludes the idea of expanded states of consciousness. Certainly, it allows for the possibility of greater or lesser intelligence. But it does not allow for mystical or divine insight.

Wilhelm Reich described this phenomenon in his discussion of what he called "Orgonomic Functionalism." In short, in order to investigate nature or gain knowledge, one must first rid one's self of the rationalizations and idealizations that function as defense mechanisms, protecting him from harsh facts about reality he does not want to face. This process has to come from within, or the mind will create even more and more elaborate defense mechanisms, finally ending in madness.

This process has traditionally been the purview of religion. However it has been dispensed with in the contemporary period.

We believe that Traditional Chinese Medicine is a modality that is divinely inspired by Masters, or people who have expanded levels of consciousness. As QiGong masters, perhaps even supernatural powers. These teachings have been assembled into sacred texts, such as **The Yellow Emperor's Classic**. It's not that science is not applicable to TCM. Certainly, anything can be rigorously studied.

For us it's mainly a question of the possibility of knowledge. Knowledge is possible as a result of divine insight. Science, however is incapable of producing positive knowledge.

While an epistemological dissertation is beyond the scope of the present volume, we look forward in the future to providing an exhaustive treatise on the subject of TCM epistemology, upon further study of **Schleiermacher, Dilthey, Heidegger** and **Gadamer**.

It might be objected that the two major researchers referred to in this work, **Rife** and **Lakhosky**, were both scientists. While it is true that they considered themselves scientists and their work adhered to rigorously applied scientific standards, our objections to "science" still stand. While scientific knowledge in and of itself may not be possible, it is the creativity and divine insight these researchers employed in developing their treatment modalities that resulted in what we now know as Electroherbalism.

We do not believe in a "third person" reality. We can only experience the world from our own individual perspective. Therefore we offer this book to you, the reader. While we don't have much first-hand experience with all the information that we are presenting, (particularly some of the material in the Appendices,) we feel that many of these ideas work for us. It is up to you to determine if they also work for you.

As acupuncturists, we have training in electro-acupuncture. Always adhere to safety precautions and keep up with the latest developments in the field. Sometimes protocols change. This information is for educational purposes, and is not meant to diagnose disease or replace a qualified healthcare practitioner. The authors, publisher and distributor are not responsible for the outcome of your patients. The reader accepts full liability for all consequences of the use of electroherbalism and other modalities noted herein.

TABLE OF CONTENTS

-What is Electroherbalism?...1
    -Types of Machines..1
    -Electroherbalism...2
    -Harmonics...3
    -CAFL...4
    -Point Prescriptions...4
    -Operation of the Machine..5
    -Signal Variance..5
    -Wave Forms...6
    -Herxheimer Reactions...7
-Manufacturers 8
-Cautions and Contra-Indications.......................................15
-Pleomorphism..16
-Royal Raymond Rife..21
-Western Pathologies...23
-George Lakhovski..47
-Materia Medica of Frequencies...49
-Formula-Based Frequencies...57
    -Bai He Gu Jin Tang
    -Bai Hu Tang
    -Bai Tou Weng Tang
    -Ban Xia Bai Zhu Tian Ma Tang
    -Ban Xia Hou Po Tang
    -Ban Xia Xie Xin Tang
    -Bao He Wan
    -Ba Zheng San
    -Ba Zhen Tang
    -Bu Yang Huan Wu Tang
    -Bu Zhong Yi Qi Tang
    -Cang Er Zhi San
    -Chai Ge Jie Ji Tang
    -Chai Hu Shu Gan San
    -Chuan Xiong Cha Tiao San
    -Da Bu Yin Wan
    -Da Chai Hu Tang
    -Da Cheng Qi Tang
    -Da Jian Zhong Tang
    -Dang Gui Bu Xue Tang
    -Dang Gui Liu Huang Tang
    -Dao Chi San
    -Ding Chuan Tang

-Du Huo Ji Sheng Tang
-Du Qi Wan
-Er Chen Tang
-Er Miao San
-Er Xian Tang
-Er Zhi Wan
-Fu Yuan Huo Xue Tang
-Gan Mai Da Zao Tang
-Gan Mao Ling
-Ge Gen Huang Lian Huang Qin Tang
-Ge Gen Tang
-Ge Xia Zhu Yu Tang
-Gui Pi Tang
-Gui Zhi Shao Yao Zhi Mu Tang
-Gui Zhi Tang
-Gui Zhi Fu Ling Wan
-Huang Lian E Jiao Tang
-Huang Lian Jie Du Tang
-Huo Xiang Zheng Qi San
-Jiao Ai Tang
-Ji Chuan Jian
-Jin Gui Shen Qi Wan
-Jin Suo Gu Jing Wan
-Juan Bi Tang
-Ju Pi Zhu Ru Tang
-Ling Gui Zhu Gan Tang
-Ling Jiao Gou Teng Tang
-Liu Wei Di Huang Wan
-Li Zhong Wan
-Long Dan Xie Gan Tang
-Ma Huang Tang
-Mai Men Dong Tang
-Ma Xing Shi Gan Tang
-Ma Xing Yi Gan Tang
-Ma Zi Ren Wan
-Mu Li San
-Nuan Gan Jian
-Ping Wei San
-Pu Ji Xiao Du Yin
-Qiang Huo Sheng Shi Tang
-Qi Ju Di Huang Wan
-Qing Gu San
-Qing Hao Bie Jia Tang
-Qing Qi Hua Tan Wan

-Qing Wei San
-Qing Ying Tang
-Qing Zao Jiu Fei Tang
-Ren Shen Bai Du San
-Sang Ju Yin
-Sang Piao Xiao San
-Sang Xing Tang
-San Zi Yang Qin Tang
-Shao Fu Zhu Yu Tang
-Shao Yao Tang
-Sheng Hua Tang
-Sheng Mai San
-Shen Ling Bai Zhu San
-Shen Tong Zhu Yu Tang
-Shi Quan Da Bu Tang
-Shi Xiao San
-Si Jun Zi Tang
-Si Ni San
-Si Shen Wan
-Si Wu Tang
-Suan Zao Ren Tang
-Su Zi Jiang Qi Tang
-Tian Ma Gou Teng Yin
-Tian Tai Wu Yao San
-Tian Wang Bu Xin Dan
-Tiao Wei Cheng Qi Tang
-Tong Xie Yao Fang
-Wan Dai Tang
-Wen Dan Tang
-Wen Jing Tang
-Wu Ling San
-Wu Pi San
-Wu Wei Xiao Du Yin
-Wu Zhu Yu Tang
-Xiao Chai Hu Tang
-Xiao Cheng Qi Tang
-Xiao Feng San
-Xiao Jian Zhong Tang
-Xiao Qing Long Tang
-Xiao Yao San
-Xie Bai San
-Xie Xin Tang
-Xi Jiao Di Huang Tang
-Xing Su San

-*Xue Fu Zhu Yu Tang*
-*Yi Guan Jian*
-*Yin Chen Hao Tang*
-*Yin Qiao San*
-*You Gui Wan*
-*You Gui Yin*
-*Yue Ju Wan*
-*Yu Nu Jian*
-*Yu Ping Feng San*
-*Zhen Gan Xi Feng Tang*
-*Zhen Wu Tang*
-*Zhi Bai Di Huang Tang*
-*Zhi Gan Cao Tang*
-*Zhi Sou San*
-*Zhu Ling Tang*
-*Zhu Ye Shi Gao Tang*
-*Zou Gui Wan*
-*Zuo Jin Wan*

APPENDICES

-Beck Protocols...191
    -Magnetic Pulser...191
    -Blood Electrification..192
    -Ozone Water...192
    -Colloidal Silver..193
    -Silver Pulser..194
    -Argyria: Chelation Protocols...............................195
-Hulda Clark..197
    -Zapper..197
    -Syncrometer..197
    -Green Black Walnut Tincture................................198
-Microelectricitygermkiller..199
    -Godzilla...200
    -GodRods..200
-SCENAR...202
-MRSA..203
-Harmonics..208
    -Wave Harmonics...208
    -Function Harmonics..208
-Novobiotronics...209
-BIBLIOGRAPHY..210

THE USE OF ELECTROHERBALISM IN TRADITIONAL CHINESE MEDICINE

Electroherbalism is the same thing as electro-acupuncture. The only difference is that you're using targeted frequencies for specific therapeutic purposes. For this reason, specialized technology is required.

Types of Machines

There are two main types of frequency generators in Electroherbalism. The first is the electrical contact pad device. This type of device consists of the frequency generator, then includes metallic hand tubes and foot plates. The user selects which he wants to use. He can stand on the metallic foot plates or hold the tubes in his hands. This is how the frequencies are passed into the body, using the medium of electricity.

We convert these machines for use in electro-acupuncture. Nowadays these machines commonly come from the manufacturer with TENS electrodes, which fit perfectly on acupuncture points. Barring this, we will take the wires that attach to the foot plates and connect them to acupuncture needles using alligator clips.

The second type of machine is the plasma tube device. These devices use glass tubes filled with noble gasses, the contents of which differ from researcher to researcher and manufacturer to manufacturer, to broadcast the signal into the patient's body. The advantage of these machines is that the patient does not have to be in physical contact with the bulb. The disadvantage is that these machines tend to be far more expensive than contact pad devices.

There is one other device that uses an electromagnetic coil. This is called the "Doug Coil." We will describe this machine later. It is not produced by manufacturers, but the schematics are available online. It is very popular with people who use electroherbalism to treat Lyme's Disease.

So you go through the normal process of electro-acupuncture, only you set the machine to run each frequency for a minimum of 3-5 minutes. You might also prefer to use TENS pads rather than needles to electrify the points. In fact, you could also use a plasma tube, foot plates or hand tubes, although people usually stand on the foot plates.

Electroherbalism

First of all, what we have done is that we have focused on **George Lakhovsky** over **Royal Raymond Rife**. **Rife** is so central to the Western practice of electroherbalism, that it's often just called "Rife" for short. **Rife** was great. His idea was to kill germs using frequencies. **Lakhovsky**'s idea was to strengthen the normal functioning of healthy cells. Therefore, we differentiate between "Rife" and "electroherbalism," strictly speaking. For us, "Rife" alludes to the Western application of killing pathogens, whereas "electroherbalism" can refer to either the killing of pathogens OR the strengthening of healthy cells. But we usually mean the latter.

TCM has a different medical ontology than Western medicine. There is not the same type of "germ theory" per se in TCM. As a matter of fact, even in Rife/electroherbalism, there is a different form of the "germ theory." The generally accepted paradigm in electroherbalism and Rife therapy is that of pleomorphism. We will get more into that later, as it has some unique similarities with TCM. But generally, TCM is more concerned with the function of subtle energies.

The first thing we had to do was to convert the functions and indications of the frequencies into the language of TCM. This was no small task, and as you can imagine, required a certain level of interpretation and subjectivity. We focused mainly on the **Lakhovsky** type frequencies. We created lists of frequencies, based upon their Western functions and indications, interpreted from a TCM standpoint. Then we selected the most commonly occurring frequencies for each function and indication. For this we used an algorithm, which weighted each frequency based on how many times it was used for different Western applications, which would have the same sort of function and indication from a TCM standpoint.

From this, we arrived at our "Materia Medica" of frequencies for each function and indication. We categorized the frequencies as Primary, Secondary and Tertiary, based upon how many different ways they were each used for each function and indication. We used the same grouping of functions and indications as we used in our book on essential oils, except that we combined "moving qi and blood" into one group. From this "Materia Medica" of frequencies, we calculated frequency lists for many of the traditional herbal formulas, using the same algorithm, weighting each frequency based upon whether each frequency was Primary, Secondary or Tertiary.

To calculate frequencies for a formula, what we did was to assemble the main functions and indications of that formula. Then we would find harmonics, or frequencies that are common to all of the functions and indications in that formula. The ones that were listed as Primary had the greatest weighting in our algorithm, the Secondary frequencies had a lesser weighting and the Tertiary the least weighting. From this we calculated a new set of Primary, Secondary and Tertiary frequencies for the overall formula.

Harmonics

To calculate harmonics, you need to calculate the factors and coefficients of the actual frequencies, in order to find numbers in common. This can be important in certain cases. For example, 27735768 Hertz is one frequency that is useful in Lyme's Disease. Many frequency generators don't go that high. So what you can do is divide in half.

As an easier illustration, let's say you want to create a wavelength 10 meters long. But your frequency generator won't go that high. What you can do is create a wave that is 5 meters long. This 5 meter wave will form a harmonic with the 10 meter wave, it will merely require two full waves to hit that same length. But the two will resonate. In these cases, it is generally recommended to run the frequency for twice as long as would normally be the case. Normally, each frequency will be run for 3-5 minutes. Each machine is designed in slightly different ways. Ours run off of software on our computers. So we will program each frequency to run for 3-5 minutes. But in a case like this, we will set it up so that this frequency will run from 6-10 minutes.

What we have done with these formulas, however, is found "harmonic" frequencies that have multiple functions and indications. We call these "function harmonics." Rather than calculate factors and coefficients, we find specific frequencies that perform multiple functions. Therefore we use one frequency to perform two or more functions simultaneously. Matching these functions and indications to acupuncture points, we calculated sets of frequencies based on the traditional Chinese herbal formulas.

Using the algorithm described earlier, we calculated sets of frequencies which are categorized into Primary, Secondary and Tertiary groups. We were very lucky, because we ended up not having to calculate any of the factors or coefficients for any of the frequencies. In each case, there were sufficient harmonics between the functions and indications required to reproduce those of the traditional herbal formulas.

CAFL

All of our frequencies are listed in Hertz and come from the CAFL. This is the standard list of frequencies, which is located at:

http://www.electroherbalism.com/Bioelectronics/FrequenciesandAnecdotes/CAFL.htm

It should be noted that there are other frequencies and other frequency lists. Many manufacturers will have their own frequency lists. Perhaps the best and most comprehensive list is in **Nenah Sylver's** book **Handbook of Rife Frequency Medicine**. We cannot recommend this book strongly enough.

Point Prescriptions

For each formula-based set of frequencies, we selected two points. These prescriptions are not etched in stone. In fact, neither are the frequencies themselves. These are just the frequency lists that we calculated, and which work for us. Our goal here is to lay out the way we do things. There has been a great deal of curiosity, so we decided to share the way we do it with all of you.

We will generally use Jia Ji points if possible. We use DU 14 quite a bit. We also prefer Yuan Source points. This is because we are generally treating yin organs. For yang organs we will use Front Mu and Lower He Sea points. So to some degree it depends what you are treating. Match the functions and indications of the frequencies to those of the points.

Operation of the Machine

All machines are designed somewhat differently. Ours are run from software on a computer. What you want to do is the same thing as you would do in a normal electro-acupuncture treatment. Make sure the patient is comfortable and insert the needles. Then use alligator clamps to attach the wires to the needles in the points you want to treat. Alternatively, you can use TENS electrodes. These are sticky electrically conductive electrodes which attach to the body. We have found that they give a better connection than needles do, as they have more surface area. Needles do seem to be better at directing the qi and the electrical current, to some degree. We haven't done a formal study on this.

One thing we will sometimes do is use a water-based conductant with the TENS electrodes. We will mix a few drops of an essential oil blend with the conductant gel, then tape the electrodes over the desired point. We believe that the essential oils will boost the effect of the treatment.

Signal Variance

One feature that many machines will use is called "gating." This means that the frequency signal will be sent out in a pulse. It will run normally, then suddenly a large pulse of extra power will go through. This will not be noticeable to the patient, but it tends to knock out the few germs inside the body that are extra tough and are not being killed by the regular administration of the frequency. Each machine is programmed differently, but on ours, if we want to use the gating feature, there are commands for that in the software. It's a great feature.

Our machines actually can run THREE signals at the same time. So you have your regular frequency that is being delivered, then simultaneously you can send a pulsed signal, and underneath it all you can run a "carrier" frequency. A carrier frequency will carry the rest of the signals deeper into the body. Most machines are sufficiently powerful to kill pathogens throughout the body, although applying them only onto two points diminishes the points of contact of electrical stimulation from the entire hands or feet, which is what the machines are designed for. Still, we feel that the targeted points actually increase the efficacy of the treatment overall. And frankly, the signal is still sufficient to resonate throughout the body.

In electroherbalism, the strength of the power level is considered to be a significant factor. This is especially true if the signal needs to penetrate deeply into the body. In electro-acupuncture, it's more important for the patient to feel comfortable. You don't want to crank the power up so high that the electrical signal is actually painful. However in electroherbalism, this is slightly different. The power level DOES matter. We mitigate this by eliminating the lower frequencies. We list the frequencies in each set from lower to higher, so that the more painful frequencies are finished first. That way if the patient is uncomfortable, we can skip over them. Once the frequency gets over 4000 Hertz, you can't even feel them anymore. This is a great advantage to people who are sensitive to discomfort.

We feel that the electricity will tend to resonate with the rest of the needles that are being used in the treatment. Electricity is a "flow of electrons," which are quanta of aether or "qi." Pure energy. We feel that the electricity will boost the function of the needles in directing qi.

So the patient will be on the table, and the machine is programmed to run through a specific set of frequencies. This should be timed to coincide with the length of the treatment, but each frequency should be run for a minimum of three minutes. Each list has a different number of frequencies, but generally it's quite easy to run through them all in one treatment session. There's no need to run through all of them either.

Oftentimes, people will feel certain frequencies resonating with the condition being treated. This is most common in Western style infections. If the patient feels that a certain frequency or two is "resonating" or vibrating particularly well with an infected area, this likely means that those particular frequencies are being extra effective there. We will take note of this and use that frequency again the next time, perhaps for a longer period of time.

Wave Forms

There are two main wave forms used in Electroherbalism. These are the square wave and the sine wave. Generally, people use the square wave for killing pathogens and the sine wave for promoting health. However there is no real consensus on this. Experiment on your own, see what works for you. Square waves by their nature will tend to have more harmonics. Many machines only produce square waves. Other wave forms include triangular and sawtooth waves.

Herxheimer Reactions

After the treatment, the patient is likely to experience a Herxheimer effect. This occurs when there is a die-off of infectious pathogens, or when the qi has dislodged some sort of toxins within the body. This may cause the patient to feel a little bit sicker for a day or two. But it's actually a "healing crisis." The body is expelling the dead bodies of germs or some sort of TCM style toxin, like phlegm. Have the patient drink lots of water and get plenty of rest.

Treatments should be spaced out by approximately two to three days to enable the body to clear out the bad stuff. You do want to do at least three treatments if you're killing germs, because you want to make sure you get them all. You do not want to generate "super resistance" to your frequencies by allowing stragglers to live on. This is another reason the gating feature is important. It kills the majority of these stragglers. Electroherbalism functions in a similar way to that of antibiotics. You have to keep taking the antibiotics, even after you're no longer experiencing symptoms. This isn't as important if you're just doing a TCM based treatment. In that case, you just want the treatment to hold. They should still drink plenty of water, though.

MANUFACTURERS

Most people, when they hear about electroherbalism wonder if it's real. They suspect it's overly-hyped, but they're not sure. They may be curious, but the machines are too expensive for the risk involved, if the technology turns out to be overrated. There are less expensive options, though. There are numerous forums online, where people will sell used machines. Many times these machines are barely used and in great shape. But again, a used machine might be damaged or in sub-optimal condition.

Here is a list of manufacturers of frequency generators, in random order:

Pacific Health
http://www.pachealthonline.com/products.htm

These are the machines we use. They're not the best machines out there, but we believe they may be the best value for the money. Pacific Health sells a number of different devices in different price ranges. If you're unsure about the technology, get one of the lower end units and experiment with it. They start out around $399.00. Pacific Health also offers a plasma tube unit.

We use the programmable blaster 1.5 Hz. This uses an Atelier Robin 125, which isn't necessarily the state of the art, but it works great, and it is affordable for grad students, like us. We started out with a more basic unit, but it worked so great that we upgraded. The Atelier Robin generator runs off of a computer, with the software available from the manufacturer's website and also on a disc that come with the unit.

Learning how to program the unit is moderately difficult. This can be a turnoff to some people, because often times, people are ill, and may have "brain fog." So if you need to treat yourself without assistance, you may want to invest in a device that is simpler to use. Most of the lower end units are pretty simple to learn, but you have to dial in the frequencies individually, rather than just cutting and pasting them into software and running the whole set.

One thing about the device we use is that it is very easy to adapt for use in electro-acupuncture. As with many other machines, TENS electrodes are included, as are alligator clip connectors, which are what we use to attach them to acupuncture needles. Other machines may or may not all be as easy to modify for our purposes.

Doug Coil

http://health.groups.yahoo.com/group/qsc1850hd/

The Doug Coil device is a very popular machine that is often home-constructed. To our knowledge, it is not manufactured commercially. However, schematics for the device are posted online for free. Do not try to construct the device yourself if you lack the expertise to do so. This machine is unique in that it runs off of neither a contact pad nor a bulb, but an electromagnetic coil.

This machine is very powerful. It is a favorite for treatment of Lyme's Disease. However it can only run one frequency at a time. Shown above is an email group available for discussion of this device, although it is not very active anymore.

Wellness Pro

http://www.globalwellnesspro.com/

The Wellness Pro is another very popular machine. It is the only electroherbalism device that has been cleared by the FDA as a TENS unit for pain. This device is also quite easy to learn.

The Wellness Pro 2010 and 2013 Wellness Pro+ has 1000 Pre-programmed auto codes with the option to program up to one million different frequencies. (TENS and Micro Current) It is capable of all the standard signal variance functions and is a contact device. You may receive a discount if you go through a distributor.

Electromedical Technologies
3104 E. Camelback Road #528,
Phoenix, AZ 85016

Toll Free: (888) 880-7888
Direct: (480) 292-8976
Fax: (480) 452-1518
customercare@globalwellnesspro.com

EMEM
http://www.stenulson.net/althealth/index.htm

The EMEM device, or "Experimental Electromagnetic Machine" is a plasma tube device that may be constructed on your own or purchased commercially. Therefore the price may tend to vary. Some machines will also have a contact pad adaptability. The main types of tubes are the phanotron, which is more of a tube or a sphere, and the "double bubble." They are filled with noble gases, the content of which varies from researcher to researcher.

The EMEM device will generally have a pretty wide frequency range. It is a powerful device and has an excellent track record. Especially among the Lyme Disease community.

BCX Ultra
http://www.bioelectricsforhealth.com/

The BCX Ultra is another popular machine. It is advertised on many alternative health podcasts and radio shows. It is commercially available, and you can quite often find moderately priced used devices. These devices use both plasma tubes and contact pads, and will produce over 15 different wave forms. They also have an extremely wide frequency range in both the tube and contact pad modes. The plasma tubes are in the form of the hand tubes.

The BCX Ultra is very easy to learn. It has 1240 frequency sets automatically pre-programmed, with the ability to program your own frequency lists. It also comes with an instructional DVD.

1-800-936-6240

GB4000

http://www.thegb4000.com/

The GB4000, as many of the above is also very popular and has a following among electroherbalism users. This device comes with a plasma tube attachment. A touted feature on the GB4000 is that it can run 8 frequencies simultaneously, and has an extremely wide frequency range. It can run both square and sine waves.

Contact info:
info@thegb4000.com
877-743-3757
208-703-1604

ProWave 101

http://urparamount.com/Contact/

The ProWave 101 is another popular manufactured machine. It has a pretty good frequency range and produces a pure square wave. Its proprietary Bio-Impedance Matching technology allows the square wave to remain square through the body tissue. It has both hundreds of condition programs consisting of multiple frequencies set by the manufacturer and the ability to program your own.

These machines are also known as Rife 101 devices. They are cordless and rechargeable but may also be used plugged in. They come with the same attachments as most machines, plus flexible wristband electrodes. They also have a sensor that will tell you how well the signal is penetrating your body. For a nominal fee, this machine can be sent in for periodic software updates, ensuring it always has the latest modifications.

URparamount, Inc.
6080 Huntwick #305, Delray Beach, FL 33484
info@URparamount.com
Phone: 561-291-9780

JWLabs
www.jwlabs.com
www.rifemachine.com

John Wright has been constructing frequency generators for 27 years. He was originally approached by friends of Rife. Their original machines, "Model B," were analog machines built with vacuum tubes. They were very popular and reliable machines.

The current machine, Model A, uses a pre-recorded CD of frequency treatments, which is converted to therapeutic output. It has a very small size, and a frequency range up to 10,000 Hertz. It can run off of batteries or an AC wall plug.

JWLabs has been around for a long time, has excellent customer support and a full lifetime warranty. They train each new customer on the use of the machine, and are endorsed by the Budwig Clinic.

info@rifemachine.com
1-951-926-6415
888.891.1122

Alixxor
http://www.alixxor.com/

The Alixxor is a contact pad device that can also be used as a colloidal silver generator, a "Bob Beck" blood electrification device and a TENS device. You can use 2000 pre-programmed frequency sets or save your own. This machine has a 5 year warranty.

James Bare

http://plasmasonics.com/
http://www.rifetechnologies.com/

James Bare is a chiropractor who has been experimenting with the development of plasma tube devices for many years. We regard him as one of the primary developers of this technology.

He provides a booklet on how to build your own plasma tube device for far less money than you would spend on a commercially manufactured device. He offers a pre-assembled kit as well as parts to manufacture your own machine. **James Bare** also works with **Novobiotronics**, a non-profit research organization devoted to the development of electro-medicine.

jbare@plasmasonics.com

PERL

https://www.resonantlight.com/

Resonant Light Technology is a Canadian manufacturer of premium devices, including the ProGen II frequency generator and the PERL-M, a plasma-tube PEMF machine. The ProGen II can run the PERL, or be used with TENS pads. This company has been manufacturing these types of devices since 1996, and they are very well thought of. The units are easy to use and extremely reliable.

P: 1.250.338.4949
Toll Free US: 1.877.338.4949
F: 1.877.338.4949
info@resonantlight.com

Resonant Light Technology Inc.

4875 North Island Highway
Courtenay, BC
CANADA
V9N 5Y9

True Rife

http://www.truerife.com/

With over 1500 researchers within their network and over 20,000 instruments, Truerife is dedicated to frequency research and development. TrueRife is an International company that ships around the globe.

True Rife
564 Fineview
Kalamazoo, MI 49004
USA
truerife@truerife.com

FSCAN

http://www.fscan.com

The FSCAN produces both square and sine waves and has a wide frequency range. It is considered to be an easy machine to use, with the ability to store your own frequency sets or use sets that are pre-programmed. You can also use the USB attachment to operate it from a computer.

The most unique feature of the FSCAN is its function in scanning the body and giving you a list of frequencies to run based upon the results of that scan. No other machine has this feature.

Despite its uniqueness and the high quality of its production, the FSCAN has a number of very reasonably priced models. It is a very popular machine.

CAUTIONS AND CONTRAINDICATIONS

-Do not use a contact pad device if the patient has electrical issues with the heart, or epileptic/seizure activity.

-The use of these devices is not as strictly cautioned as electro-acupuncture devices. It is a common practice to cross the center line of the body, for instance. However we adhere to the traditional rules of electro-acupuncture as we have been taught. Therefore, rather than using the same point bilaterally, we will generally select two points on one side of the body. Always use common sense.

-Drink plenty of water before and after a treatment. When you undergo electroherbalism therapy, you may have significant die off of pathological microbes. This is known as a Herxheimer reaction, or "herxing." You need to be able to flush all these dead microbes out of your system. Anti-oxidants might help as well. Oftentimes a patient will feel slightly more ill after the treatment due to this effect, but this is normal.

-Pregnant women should not use these devices, as the effects upon the fetus are unknown. Nursing mothers also should not use the device, due to the Herxheimer effect, which may pollute her milk.

-The devices should also not be used on infants.

-Do not use these devices on transplantees.

-Do not use the machine if your body is too weak to handle the Herxheimer effect.

-It is important to make sure you have killed all the germs, if that is what you are using it for. Do at least 2-3 treatments. Electroherbalism works on a similar principle to that of antibiotics. It is theoretically possible that insufficient use of frequencies could generate germs that are super-resistant to the frequencies.

-Use with caution on people with metallic implants. (A sensation of heat/tingling at the site of the implant may suggest internal burning. Decrease power, change frequency, decrease time of exposure, possibly move electrodes or discontinue treatment altogether.)

PLEOMORPHISM

The generally accepted etiological paradigm in electroherbalism is that of pleomorphism. Pleomorphism represents a sort of middle ground between the conventional Western "germ theory" and that of TCM pathology. It accepts the Western concepts of "germs," but it gives an alternative thesis as to their presence in the body.

The conventional "germ theory" holds that germs attack the body from the outside. They must come from an external source and contaminate the body by various routes. These germs can mutate from time to time, but this is no different than the normal course of Darwinian evolution, and results from random mutations which happen to be more adaptive to the environment.

Pleomorphism holds that germs spontaneously generate from normal cells from inside the body. Some theorists claim that they spontaneously form from nano bits called "protits" or "bions" or "microzymas." Others claim that they pleomorph from normal intestinal bacteria or other cells.

Our original plan for this book was to focus on Pleomorphism, from the standpoint of TCM. We believe that TCM pathology could go a long way to explain (and predict) the phenomena of pleomorphism. The two systems of pathology are hardly mutually exclusive.

We are all familiar, as TCM practitioners, with the theories of pathology. The six evils. The 5 element cycle. According to the Western theory of pleomorphism, there are other, but perhaps related factors.

According to this theory, the body remains healthy as long as it is maintained by sufficient nutrition. However, when there is a disharmony, illness may set in. There are a number of factors that may contribute to this condition:

1: **Malnutrition.** This is particularly of concern nowadays with GM crops and processed foods which contain little if any nutrition.

2: **Toxicity.** This may include everything from pharmaceuticals to impurities in foods, EMF fields, to sleep deprivation.

3: **Acid/Alkaline balance in the body.** The ideal pH for the blood is generally considered to be somewhere from about 7.35-7.5. Outside of this general range, the body may become ill.

4: **Proliferation of pathogenic microbes.** Generally "germs" thrive in an acidic environment. This is true of bacteria, fungi, viruses and parasites alike. Oxygen deficiency can play a part here too, because most pathogens do very well in an anaerobic environment. These pathogens not only feed on the diseased bodily tissues, but excrete wastes into the environment as well.

5: **Positive mental attitude**. If a person is depressed or has a negative or obsessive thought pattern, this can stagnate qi in the body, leading to a toxic environment for proliferation of microtoxicity.

This is not to say that germs cannot attack the body from outside. It's just saying that that is not necessarily the case.

Antoine Bechamp (1816-1908)

Antoine Bechamp was a contemporary of Pasteur. His scientific resume included a degree as Doctor of Medicine, Doctor of Science, Master of Pharmacy, Professor of Medical Chemistry and Pharmacy, Professor of Biological Chemistry, Fellow and Professor of Physics and Toxicology and Dean of the Free Faculty of Medicine at the University of Lille, France.

Bechamp found that living cells were made up of smaller, more basic units he called "microzymas." These microzymas promote the transformation of living tissue through the process of nutrition. In healthy cells, they would be responsible for forming cellular tissue.

The problem is that, in a toxic environment, they would form into pathogens. These pathogenic microbes can form any of several different types, chief among them being bacteria, viruses and fungi. (Bacteria are thought to be the first type of pathogens to form during this process.) These pathogenic microbes function to break down and ferment tissue that is already sick.

For instance in TCM we might say that there is not enough qi to support the continued life functioning of the tissue. So the pathogenic microbes break it down into more basic chemical elements though putrefaction. When this process is finished, the microzymas go back to their original non-pathogenic form.

The body remains healthy as long as it is maintained by sufficient nutrition or qi. However, when there is a disharmony, illness may set in.

Günther Enderlein (1872 – 1968)

German scientist **Guenther Enderlein** believed that the life cycle of micro-organisms included the ability to take on more complex lifeforms with increased functionality as a result. He differentiated this from the normal process of "mutation" theorized about in biological evolution. He called these fundamental organisms "endobions," and he wrote about them in **The Life Cycle of Bacteria**. **Enderlein** coined the term "pleomorphism."

Enderlein did not believe that any bacteria could pleomorph into just any other bacteria, virus or fungus. Each type was strictly limited as to the type of pathogens into which it could pleomorph. However, he believed that this pleomorphism was part of the normal cycle of cellular growth and development. He developed his own remedies which are still sold today through the company he founded, Sanum-Kehlbeck.

Edward Rosenow (1875-1966)

Dr. Edward Rosenow spent 60 years with the Mayo Clinic and published hundreds of articles in medical journals. In one article, published in the Journal of Infectious Diseases, he claimed that the streptococcus that invades the throat and the pneumococcus that invades the lungs are actually the same bacteria, which pleomorphs, based upon the different types of tissue off of which it is feeding.

Wilhelm Reich (1897 – 1957)

Wilhelm Reich, in **Bion Experiments on the Orgins of Life** referred to these microzymas/endobions/protits as "bions." **Reich** was a very prolific, albeit non-mainstream researcher. In addition to finding a somatic basis for psychoanalysis and positing an "aether physics" theory, he also devoloped evidence for abiogenesis. This is similar to pleomorphism, except that it goes even farther, to posit outright spontaneous generation.

Lida Mattman (1912 – 2008)

Lida Mattman was a renowned member of the American Society for Microbiology and the Michigan Academy of Science. She wrote a book called **Stealth Pathogens: Cell Wall Deficient Forms**. She did alot of work on Lyme's Disease. There is a great Youtube video of her speaking on stealth pathogens at an Autoimmunity Research Foundation conference in Chicago from 2005.

Gaston Naessens (1924 – Present)

Naessens created his own super-powerful microscope, which he calls a Somatoscope. He calls the microzymas/endobions/protits/bions "somatids." **Naessens** was involved in some controversy in Canada during the 1990s for his theories of pleomorphism. **Christopher Bird** wrote a book about it called, **The Persecution and Trial of Gaston Naessens.**

Others

Other researchers include **Virginia Livingston-Wheeler, Eleanor Alexander-Jackson, Irene Diller, Florence Seibert, Alan Cantwell**, and many others. **Nenah Sylver** goes much deeper on pleomorphism in her excellent book, **Rife Handbook of Frequency Therapy**. We highly recommend Nenah's book. We wanted to touch on this topic, as it is important, however our main focus in this book is to give the basics of how to perform electroherbalism treatments, from the standpoint of TCM.

ROYAL RAYMOND RIFE

The traditional forefather of electroherbalism is commonly thought of as being **Royal Raymond Rife**. This is so much the case, that even today, many people refer to the technology as "Rife Technology," and to people who utilize the technology as "Rifers." As we have stated previously, **Rife** developed the conventional "Western" approach to using frequencies, to kill pathogens.

Rife was a great inventor, in the tradition of Thomas Edison and Nicola Tesla. In fact, he was their late contemporary. **Rife**'s first great invention was called the Universal Microscope. **Rife**'s microscopes were said to be so powerful, that they enabled the visual inspection of viruses. Even nowadays, this is impossible, without an electron microscope. But **Rife**'s microscope was said to be able to see the viruses in their living state.

The Universal Microscope functioned by illuminating bacteria (or whatever it was that you were looking at) based on its color. **Rife** would tune the instrument in, based upon the frequency of the light waves that would illuminate his target. From this, he concluded that it might be possible to destroy pathological microbes using frequencies as well. He spent the better part of two decades painstakingly looking through his microscope, exposing microbes to frequencies, until he found frequencies that would destroy the pathogens. He called this their "Mortal Oscillatory Rate."

The result of this research was that **Rife** had the ability to destroy pathogenic microbes in vivo, without harming the surrounding tissue. This was due to the fact that the Mortal Oscillatory Rate or MOR, was specific to the pathogen. MOR frequencies would not harm normal body cells.

The device **Rife** invented to convey the frequencies into the body was called the "Beam Ray." No one today really knows the specifics of how it worked, (not unlike the Universal Microscopes,) because unfortunately the technology was lost. However, we do know that it was more like what we use today in the form of plasma tube devices. You did not have to have physical contact with the machine in order for it to work.

Rife did develop contact pads later in his career, but he was never able to market them successfully. He had won a court case with the AMA, but his business had gone bankrupt and he was financially ruined. All in all the technology was lost, as all focus in the 1940s was moved to the newly emerging field of antibiotics.

For a much more detailed overview of **Rife**'s life and work, see **Nenah Sylver's Rife Handbook of Frequency Therapy and Holistic Health**. Our purpose here is to just give a brief overview of **Rife** and his work, so that a person can understand the basics enough to get started using the technology.

Western Diagnoses

NOTE: These frequencies are suggested for patients who have Western Diagnoses. They are not meant to be the sole treatment modality, but to be used in conjunction with herbs, acupuncture and also in conjunction with the patient's Western physician.

As always, our frequencies are derived from the CAFL, which exists at the following link:

http://www.electroherbalism.com/Bioelectronics/FrequenciesandAnecd otes/CAFL.htm

Each frequency should be applied for a minimum of 3-5 minutes. We list our frequency sets from lower to higher. This allows us to skip over the lower frequencies straight to the higher, in cases in which patients might find the lower frequencies to be uncomfortable. All frequencies are in Hertz.

For other frequency lists, consult the various manufacturers of electroherbalism machines. Many of the manufacturers will have their own frequency lists. See also **Nenah Sylver's** excellent **Rife Handbook of Frequency Therapy.**

Acne

Acne (run 564 for 6 min) - 2720, 2170, 1800, 1600, 1550, 1552, 1500, 802, 880, 778, 787, 760, 741, 727, 660, 564, 465, 450, 444, 428

Suggested points:
LI 4
LU 7

Aspergillus

Aspergillus_flavus (mold found on corn, peanuts, and grain that produces aflatoxin) - 1823, 247, 1972
Aspergillus_general - 1972, 1823, 758, 743, 697, 524, 374, 339, 247
Aspergillus_glaucus (blue mold occurring in some human infectious processes) - 524, 758
Aspergillus_niger (common mold that may produce severe and persistent infection) - 374, 697
Aspergillus_terreus (mold occasionally associated with infection of the bronchi and lungs) - 743, 339

Suggested points:
Ren 12
ST 25
or
Jia Ji of UB 13
Jia Ji of UB 17

Athlete's Foot

Athletes_foot (also see Epidermophyton floccinum, Tinea, and Trichophyton rubrum freqs. Use all freqs for 5 min) - 20, 379, 727, 787, 880, 5000, 644, 766, 464, 802, 1552, 9999, 752, 923, 3176, 304

Suggested points:
SP 3
K1

Bronchitis

Bronchitis - 7344, 3672, 1234, 880, 743, 727, 683, 464, 452, 333, 72, 20, 9.39, 9.35
Bronchitis_secondary - 776, 766, 688

Suggested points:
LU 7
Ren 17

Candida Albicans

Candida_1 - 10000, 5000, 3176, 2489, 1395, 1276, 1160, 1044, 928, 877, 812, 728, 696, 580, 465, 464, 381, 348, 232, 116, 58, 20
Candida_2 (includes candida carcinomas and tropicalis) - 1403, 675, 709, 2167, 2128, 2182, 465, 20, 60, 95, 125, 225, 427, 464, 727
Candida_albicans_HC – 19217.81, 956.80
Candida_secondary (also use other parasite sets esp roundworm freqs if necessary) - 72, 422, 582, 727, 787, 802, 1016, 1134, 1153, 1550, 2222, 412, 543, 2128
Candida_sweep_TR (sweep from 12006.25 to 12137.5 by .03125 dwell 0.5 pulse 64 75)
Candida_tertiary (some causal factors) - 880, 95, 125, 20, 60, 225, 427, 240, 650, 688, 152, 442, 8146, 751, 114

Other: Hulda Clark zappers are said to be effective against Candida Albicans.

Suggested points:
ST 25, Bilateral

Chicken Pox

Chicken_pox (by the time pox marks appear, the illness is resolved and the toxins are being expelled through the skin, so must be used in the early stages of flu like symptoms after exposure. Use herpes zoster.)

Herpes_zoster (chicken pox, shingles. 664*) - 3343, 2320, 2170, 1600, 1500, 1160, 914, 880, 833, 802, 787, 664, 580, 3.9

Herpes_zoster_1 (4 min each freq) - 10000, 833, 802, 3.9

Herpes_zoster_secondary - 1550, 802, 1800, 1865, 728, 2720, 2128, 5000, 464, 800, 574, 1557, 304, 20

Herpes_zoster_v - 7160, 3343, 2431, 2323, 1577, 1544, 40887, 958, 934, 787, 786, 738, 718, 716, 686, 668, 643, 576, 574, 573, 572, 563, 554, 542, 453, 446, 436, 425, 423, 411, 345, 333, 223, 134

Suggested Points:
Du 14
Jia Ji of UB 13

Chlamydia

Chlamydia_general - 3773, 3768, 2223, 2218, 2213, 942, 866, 840, 622, 555, 470, 430

Chlamydia_pneumoniae – 7543.4, 7520.5, 4710.5, 3773.3, 3760.3, 1886, 1880, 943.3, 940, 620, 479, 471.66, 470.9, 941.8, 3767.3

Chlamydia_trachomatis (a usually sexually transmitted bacterial infection causing trachoma, inclusion conjunctivitis, lymphogranuloma venereum, urethritis, and proctitis.) - 430, 620, 624, 840, 1111.4, 2213, 866, 555.7, 2222.8

Chlamydia_trachomatis_HC – 18968.87, 944.40

Suggested points:
Liver 12, Bilateral

Cholera

Cholera (an extremely contagious and serious bacterial infection of the small intestines) - 1035, 968, 961, 851, 844, 843, 691, 591, 556, 330

Cholera_secondary - 880, 802, 450, 832, 787, 727

Suggested points:
ST 25, Bilateral

Cold, Head/Chest

Cold_1 (use 800 and 880 for 10 min, others for 5 min) - 5500, 4400, 802, 787, 727, 720, 552, 440, 400, 125, 72, 800, 880

Cold_2 - 652, 725, 746, 751, 768, 1110, 333, 666, 542, 522

Cold_3 (fall, 99. Use all freqs 5 min) - 20, 120, 146, 440, 444, 465, 727, 776, 787, 880, 1500, 1550, 5000, 1000

Cold_4 (use 880 and 800 for 10 min, 728 for 5 min) - 3176, 2489, 880, 800, 728

Cold_5 (use 7728 and 4888 for 10 min) - 7728, 4888, 8238, 2413, 880, 787, 776, 727, 440, 746, 567, 7880, 787, 300, 310, 1234, 9999

Cold_6 - 7660, 7344, 5000, 3702, 3672, 2688, 2400, 1862, 1550, 1238, 1234, 1200, 975, 880, 802, 787, 780, 778, 776, 774, 772, 770, 768, 766, 727, 688, 683, 660, 450, 412, 352

Cold_and_Flu (fall, 98. Use 8700 and 7760 for 15 min, others for 5 min) - 250, 465, 8210, 8700, 7760

Cold_and_flu_winter_01 - 959, 962

Cold_in_head_chest (Mutates constantly; too many strains to include complete list of frequencies. See also Strep Pneumonia, Adenovirus, Rhinitis, Coronavirus, Sinusitis, Pneumonia, Chest infection, and Rhino pneumonitis sets. Use lots of echinacea at onset to prevent cell damage that prolongs healing,even if correct freqs are found.) - 10000, 7344, 4412, 3176, 2489, 1550, 880, 802, 787, 776, 766, 728, 712, 688, 683, 665, 660, 600, 444, 333, 20

Cold_2005_TR – 10000, 7344, 5000, 2950, 2900, 2650, 2600, 1550, 1234, 740, 880, 787, 727, 330, 165, 82.6, 41.75, 20.87, 30

Suggested points:
Jia Ji of UB 13
DU 14

Conjunctivitis

Conjunctivitis (also known as pink eye. Also use Chlamydia trachomatis and see Bacillus subtilis if necessary) - 2025, 1830, 1552, 1550, 1246, 1206, 880, 822, 802, 787, 727, 722, 489, 432, 80, 20

Suggested points:
Taiyang
GB 14

Cryptosporidium

Cryptosporidium (parasitic protozoa sometimes causing diarrhea in humans) - 220, 482, 575, 4122, 698, 711, 893, 895, 1276, 5690

Suggested points:
ST 25, Bilateral

Dental Infections

Dental_and_jawbone_infections_1 (use converge 1 1 on all except use converge 1 0.1 on 728) - 7270, 2720, 2170, 880, 787, 727, 500, 190, 728
Dental_and_jawbone_infections_2 – 15, 326, 465, 727, 787, 880
Dental_foci (Neglecting this can prevent recovery from any illness if infection is a problem) - 5170, 3000, 2720, 2489, 1800, 1600, 1550, 1500, 880, 832, 802, 787, 776, 727, 666, 650, 646, 600, 465, 190, 95, 47.5
Dental_general (see also Toothache) - 728, 784, 635, 640, 1036, 1043, 1094, 685, 60, 48, 465
Dental_infection (roots and gums) - 960, 660, 666, 690, 727, 784, 787, 800, 880, 1560, 1840, 1998, 2489
Dental_infection_1 - 5170, 3000, 2720, 2489, 1800, 1600, 1550, 1500, 1094, 1043, 1036, 880, 832, 802, 787, 776, 727, 685, 666, 650, 646, 640, 635, 600, 465, 190, 95, 60, 48, 47.5
Dental_infection_2 - 10000, 5000, 1562, 1552, 1550, 880, 800, 799, 787, 784, 776, 774, 728, 727, 664, 620, 464, 254.2, 120, 64, 20
Dental_infection_and_Earache_1 - 960, 930, 900, 880, 832, 802, 800, 787, 776, 775, 768, 760, 750, 727, 685, 680, 666, 650, 646.3, 646, 640, 635, 622.3, 547, 521, 518
Dental_infections_TR – 3400, 2489, 1700, 1560
Dental_Infections_v - 981, 138, 142, 177, 183, 210, 222, 233, 436, 534, 626, 723, 835, 875, 5227, 7059
Toothache (to neglect this can prevent recovery from any illness. Should also be treated professionally. See also Dental, Dental foci, Gingivitis, Pyorrhea.) - 5170, 3000, 2720, 2489, 1800, 1600, 1550, 1500, 880, 832, 802, 787, 776, 776, 727, 666, 650, 646, 600, 465, 190, 95, 47.5

The Godzilla is said to be very effective in these cases.

Suggested points:
Ren 23
ST 6

Dysentery

Dysentery (acute diarrhea with blood and mucus. Also use Entamoeba histolytica, Salmonella, and Shigella) - 1552, 802, 832

Entamoeba_histolytica (highly damaging protozoa causing dysentery and liver infection) - 148, 166, 308, 393, 631, 778

Entamoeba_histolytica_HC - 19168.02, 954.32

Entamoeba_histolytica_secondary – 1552, 880, 802, 1550, 832, 787, 727, 690, 660, 465, 786, 768, 523, 333

Salmonella (1) - 718.2, 713.3

Salmonella (can cause intestinal inflammation and infection, and contribute to flu in children) - 1522, 718, 717, 713, 972, 664, 643

Salmonella_comp - 8656, 7771, 6787, 1634, 1522, 1244, 972, 773, 762, 754, 752, 719, 718.2, 717,713.3, 711, 707, 693, 664, 643, 546, 420, 165, 92, 59

Salmonella_enteriditis_HC (causes intestinal infection) – 16379.95, 815.51

Salmonella_paratyphi_B - 59, 92, 643, 707, 717, 719, 752, 972, 7771, 1244, 6787, 165, 711

Salmonella_paratyphi_HC – 18321.64, 912.18

Salmonella_type_B - 546, 1634

Salmonella_typhi (can cause typhoid fever) - 420, 664, 8656, 773

Salmonella_typhimurium - 693, 754, 762

Salmonella_typhimurium_HC (can cause food poisoning, nervousness, apathy) – 19168.02, 19217.81, 954.32, 956.80

Shigella (can cause acute dysentery and diarrhea as well as infect nerves, brain, and spinal cord chronically) - 621, 762, 769, 770, 1550, 802, 832

Shigella_dysenteriae_HC – 19421.39, 966.93

Suggested Points:
ST 25
ST 37

E Coli

E_coli (Escherichia coli; can cause infections in wounds and the urinary tract. If using these leads to common cold symptoms, follow with Adenovirus freqs, 800/802*, 1550/1552*) - 7849, 7847, 1730, 1722, 1552, 1550, 1320, 1244, 1000, 957, 934, 856, 840, 832, 804, 802, 800, 799, 776, 642, 634, 556, 548, 413, 333, 330, 327, 289, 282
E_coli_1 (recommended for cancer adjunct) - 7847, 1730, 1712, 1244, 1000, 934, 856, 840, 800, 776, 642, 634, 556, 539, 358, 330
E_coli_comp - 7849, 7847, 1730, 1722, 1712, 1703, 1552, 1550, 1320, 1244, 1242, 1000, 957, 934, 856, 840, 832, 804, 802, 800, 799, 776, 642, 634, 632, 556, 548, 539, 413, 358, 333, 330, 327, 289, 282E_coli_HC – 17724.20, 19566.32, 974.15, 882.44
E_coli_mutant_strain - 556, 934, 1242, 1244, 1703, 632, 634, 776

Suggested points:
ST 25
Ren 12

Eczema

Eczema - 9.19, 707, 1550, 802, 787, 727, 10000, 5000, 2720, 2008, 2180, 2128, 664, 120, 20
Eczema_1 - 770, 916, 415
Eczema_2 - 730.2, 1550, 802, 787, 690
Eczema_vascular_and_lung_disturbances – 9.39

Hulda Clark zappers may be indicated here.

Suggested points:
Ashi

Fungus, General

Fungus_and_mold_v - 4442, 2411, 1833, 1823, 1333, 1155, 1130, 1016, 942, 933, 886, 880, 866, 784, 774, 766, 745, 743, 728, 623, 623, 594, 592, 565, 555, 524, 512, 464, 414, 374, 344, 337, 321, 254, 242, 222, 158, 132
Fungus_EW_range - 823, 824, 825, 826, 827, 828, 829
Fungus_flora_1 - 331, 336, 555, 587, 632, 688, 757, 882, 884, 887
Fungus_foot_and_general_1(use 1550 for 30min) - 1550
Fungus_general (also see candida, yeast, and other specific types) - 2222, 1552, 1550, 1153, 1134, 1016, 880, 802, 787, 784, 727, 582, 465, 422, 254, 72, 20

Hulda Clark zappers are suggested.

Suggested points:
Ashi

Giardia

Giardia (use Parasites, giardia)
Parasites_general_1 - 4412, 2400, 2112, 1862, 1550, 800, 732, 728, 712, 688, 676, 644, 422, 128, 120
Parasites_general_2 - 10000, 3176, 1998, 1865, 1840, 880, 800, 780, 770, 740, 728, 727, 690, 665, 660, 465, 444, 440, 125, 120, 95, 80, 72, 47
Parasites_general_alternative_v - 4122, 1522, 967, 942, 854, 829, 827, 749, 741, 732, 633, 605, 604, 591, 524, 422, 411, 344, 172, 102
Parasites_general_comprehensive - 10000, 5000, 4412, 2720, 2400, 2112, 1864, 1550, 1360, 880, 854, 800, 784, 751, 732, 728, 712, 688, 651, 644, 524, 465, 442, 422, 334, 240, 152, 128, 125, 120, 112, 96, 72, 64, 20
Parasites_general_short_set - 20, 64, 72, 96, 112, 120, 152, 651, 732, 1360, 2720, 10000
Parasites_gen_custom2_TR (sweep 2000 to 2008 by 1 dwell 360) – 6578, 2000, 831, 2000, 2008, 2520, 689, 750, 880, 650, 187
Parasites_giardia - 5768, 5429, 4334, 2163, 2018, 1442, 829, 812, 721, 407, 334
Parasites_giardia_lamblia_HC - 21109.72, 1050.99

Suggested Points:
ST 25
ST 37

Gonorrhea

Gonorrhea - 7120, 6000, 2330, 1500, 712, 660, 600, 233, 150
Gonorrhea_neisseria_HC – 16628.88, 927.90

Suggested points:
Liver 12, bilateral

Hepatitis

Hepatitis_A (add Hepatitis general freqs if necessary) - 321, 346, 414, 423, 487, 558, 578, 693, 786, 878, 3220, 717
Hepatitis_B (add Hepatitis general freqs if necessary) - 334, 433, 767, 869, 876, 477, 574, 752, 779
Hepatitis_B_HC (antigen) – 20562.06, 1023.72
Hepatitis_C (also try Parasites, schistosoma mansoni and Hepatitis general freqs if necessary) – 5000, 3220, 3176, 2489, 2189, 1865, 1600, 1550, 1500, 1371, 933, 931, 929, 880, 802, 665, 650, 633, 625, 528, 444, 329, 317, 250, 224, 166, 146, 125, 95, 72, 28, 20
Hepatitis_C_1 - 10000, 5000, 3220, 3176, 2489, 1865, 1600, 1550, 1500, 880, 802, 665, 650, 600, 444, 250, 166, 146, 125, 95, 72, 28, 20
Hepatitis_C_TR – 728, 166, 224, 317, 727, 787, 880, 2189
Hepatitis_general - 1550, 1351, 922, 880, 802, 727, 477, 329, 317, 224, 28
Hepatitis_general_secondary - 284, 458, 477, 534, 788, 922, 9670, 768, 777, 1041
Hepatitis_general_v - 987, 934, 922, 878, 876, 842, 786, 781, 563, 562, 558, 534, 528, 477, 334, 321, 317, 224, 213, 166

Other: Beck Protocols are said to be effective against this condition, particularly in its chronic phase. The use of the magnetic pulser is encouraged in particular.

Suggested points:
Jia Ji of UB 18
LIV 3

Herpes

Herpes_general (use 1488 and 2950 for 15min, 1488*) - 2950, 1900, 1577, 1550, 1489, 1488, 629, 464, 450, 383, 304, 165, 141

Herpes_general_secondary - 37000Herpes_general_v - 165, 141, 383, 450, 629

Herpes_progenetalis (genital. Also use Herpes simplex II) - 141, 878, 898, 5310, 440, 171, 660, 590, 1175

Herpes_simplex_I (secondary. Cold sores: primarily non-genital, first try Herpes,general) - 322, 476, 589, 664, 785, 822, 895, 944, 1043, 1614, 2062, 1489, 2950

Herpes_simplex_I_1 - 339, 343, 480, 591, 778, 782, 843, 1614, 657, 699, 700, 734

Herpes_simplex_I_2 - 2489, 1800, 465, 1550, 1500, 880, 787, 727, 1850, 428

Herpes_simplex_I_3 - 470, 647, 648, 650, 652, 654, 656, 658, 660, 847, 5641, 8650

Herpes_simplex_I_4 (use 2950 for 20min) – 2950

Herpes_simplex_I_HC – 14537.82, 17201.43, 723.80, 856.41

Herpes_simplex_II - 556, 832

Herpes_simplex_II_HC – 17923.34, 17674.41, 892.35, 879.96

Herpes_simplex_IU2 – 808

Herpes_simplex_RTI (based on Resonant Light Technology's herpes set, most frequencies contracting spread. Also can be used for measles, chicken and small pox, mononucleosis, shingles, rubella, cold sores, epstein barr, variola, stoma stomatosis, and pyorrhea.) - 10000, 5000, 3176, 2489, 186, 372, 427, 446, 465, 484, 503, 522, 541, 560, 579, 598, 617, 636, 655, 674, 693, 712, 731, 750, 769, 788, 807, 826, 845, 864, 883, 902, 921, 940, 959, 978, 997, 1016, 1035, 1054, 1073, 1488, 1550, 1568, 1644, 1865, 1909, 2976, 5310, 5952

Herpes_TR (run set three times, pausing 10 minutes between runs. All frequencies can run 60 sec except 2950, which runs 180 sec) – 2950, 322, 476, 468, 589, 664, 785, 822, 895, 936, 944, 1043, 1614, 1871, 2062, 1489, 3742, 748

Herpes_type_1_anec_comp (combines most anecdotal freqs for Simplex I) - 8650, 7484, 5641, 3742, 2950, 2489, 1871, 1850, 1800, 1614, 1550, 1500, 935.5, 880, 847, 843, 787, 782, 778, 734, 727, 700, 660, 656, 652, 648, 591, 480, 467.8, 428, 343, 339

Herpes_type_2_comp - 8778, 1402, 888, 880, 848, 846, 832 , 808, 776, 732, 717, 685, 665, 556, 540, 532, 528, 373, 370, 366, 362

Herpes_type_2A - 532, 848

Herpes_type_2A_secondary - 360, 362, 364, 366, 368, 370, 373, 528, 685, 846, 880, 888, 8778, 540, 665, 716, 717, 718, 731, 732, 733, 776, 1402

Herpes_type_5 (cytomegalovirus. 2145*) - 126, 597, 629, 682, 1045, 2145, 8848, 8856
Herpes_type_C - 395, 424, 460, 533, 554, 701, 745, 2450

Other: The Beck Protocols are said to be effective against outbreaks of this condition, especially the magpulser.

Suggested points:
Jia Ji of UB 18
DU 14

Influenza

Influenza_virus_1991_1992 - 153, 345, 387, 758, 984, 985
Influenza_virus_1991_1992_secondary - 330, 332, 334, 336, 338, 340, 350, 352, 354, 356, 358, 360, 525, 632, 740, 761, 762, 776, 777, 780
Influenza_virus_1992_1993 - 535, 946
Influenza_virus_1992_1993_secondary - 272, 534, 566, 668, 674, 776, 782, 947, 632, 640, 713, 715, 742, 773, 777
Influenza_virus_1993_1994 - 757, 885, 895, 969
Influenza_virus_1993_1994_secondary - 447, 457, 597, 756, 764, 776, 798, 878, 967, 9090, 663, 720, 728, 729, 745, 762, 764, 770, 773, 779
Influenza_virus_A - 322, 332, 776
Influenza_virus_A_1974 - 442
Influenza_virus_A_Port_Chalmers - 622, 863
Influenza_virus_B - 468, 530, 532, 536, 537, 568, 722, 740, 742, 744, 746, 748, 750, 1186, 679
Influenza_virus_B_Hong_Kong - 555
Influenza_virus_British - 558, 932
Influenza_virus_general - 728, 800, 880, 7760, 8000, 8250
Influenza_virus_swine - 413, 432, 663, 839, 995
Influenza_with_Fever_v - 954, 889, 841, 787, 763, 753, 742, 523, 513, 482, 469, 461, 425, 341, 332
Influenza_with_respiratory_1 (winter 99 to 00) - 47, 1191, 2398, 2544, 5608, 7760, 7766, 672, 674, 676, 678, 680, 647, 649, 651, 653, 1215, 724, 726, 728, 730, 732, 746, 768, 687

Suggested points:
Jia Ji of UB 13
LU 7

Lyme Disease

Lyme_and_Rocky_Mtn_Spotted_Fever_v - 7989, 1590, 239, 846, 422, 417, 1455, 39975, 40439, 884, 797, 758, 693, 673, 577, 4870, 4880, 578, 128, 579

Lyme_disease (also known as borreliosis; relapsing fever in humans and animals caused by parasitic spirochetes from ticks. Also use Babesia if necessary.) - 6870, 6863, 46866, 46851, 34170, 34112, 4200, 2050, 2016, 1520, 1455, 920, 884, 800, 797, 758, 673, 625, 615, 605, 432, 345, 344, 338, 254

Lyme_1 - 864, 495, 485, 490, 495, 500, 505, 625, 610, 615, 620, 625, 630, 690, 790, 785, 790, 795

Lyme_2 (use 625 for 10 min, 615 for 5 min) - 10000, 6870, 6863, 4200, 2720, 2050, 2016, 1520, 1455, 943, 920, 885, 884, 880, 864, 800, 797, 795, 790, 785, 758, 732, 727, 699, 690, 688, 673, 664, 673, 660, 644, 630, 625, 620, 615, 610, 605, 597, 534, 533, 525, 510, 505, 495, 485, 490, 500, 484, 432, 345, 344, 338, 306, 254, 230, 3

Lyme_3 – 27735768, 1380882.58, 68750.10, 3422.87

Lyme_4 (use 2016 and 625 for 10 min, others for 5 min) - 2050, 1520, 615, 2016, 625Lyme_5 (use 920 for 10 min) - 920

Lyme_6 (borrelia afzellii) - 387500

Lyme_7 (borrelia burgdorferi) - 380000

Lyme_8 (borrelia garinii) - 382000

Lyme_hatchlings_eggs - 640, 8554, 203, 412, 414, 589, 667, 840, 1000, 1072, 1087, 1105

Lyme_JB - 27735768

Lyme_secondary (254*) - 254, 525, 597, 644, 885, 699

Lyme_tertiary - 306, 432, 484, 610, 625, 690, 864, 2016, 790

Lyme_TR_A (Program A, run every other day) – 6675, 4879, 2899, 2720, 2016, 1800, 1600, 1550, 1519, 1455, 1433, 885, 880, 863, 828, 802, 786, 776

Lyme_TR_B (Program B, run every other day) – 765, 758, 749, 726, 672, 604, 600, 581, 464, 451, 432, 345, 250, 144, 62

See also: **When Antibiotics Fail: Lyme Disease and Rife Machines** by **Bryan Rosner** et al.

Suggested Points:
Ashi

Measles

Measles - 727, 787, 880, 342, 442, 443, 467, 520, 521, 552, 1489, 745, 757, 763, 712

Measles_HC (antigen) – 18471.00, 919.62

Measles_rubella (German or 3 day measles) - 431, 459, 510, 517, 796, 967, 368, 734, 772

Measles_rubella_secondary - 727, 787, 880

Measles_rubella_vaccine - 429, 459, 832, 926, 505

Measles_rubeola (9 day measles) - 342, 467, 520, 784, 787, 962, 1489

Measles_vaccine - 214, 725, 747, 783, 962

Measles_w_vaccine - 1489, 962, 880, 787, 783, 763, 757, 747, 745, 727, 725, 712, 552, 521, 467, 443, 342, 214

Suggested points:
DU 14
Jia Ji of UB 13

Mumps

Mumps (acute viral inflammation of the saliva glands. See also Coxsackie) - 152, 242, 642, 674, 922

Mumps_HC (antigen) – 19018.66, 946.88

Mumps_secondary - 190, 235, 516, 1243, 1660, 2630, 3142, 9667, 729, 741, 759, 761, 1170

Mumps_tertiary - 10000, 727, 2720, 2489, 2127, 2008, 428, 880, 787, 727, 20

Mumps_vaccine - 273, 551, 711, 730, 1419

Suggested points:
Ren 23
ST 5

Parasites

Parasites_ancylostoma_braziliense_HC (Dog and cat hookworm, the larva of which is the most common cause of cutaneous larva migrans aka creeping eruption. Also see Parasites hookworm) - 19964.61, 993.98

Parasites_ancylostoma_caninum_HC - 19914.83, 991.50, 19566.32, 974.15, 19217.81, 956.80

Parasites_ascaris (152*) - 152, 442, 8146, 751, 1146, 797

Parasites_ascaris_HC (larvae in lung) – 20313.12, 1011.33Parasites_ascaris megalocephala_HC - 20313.12, 1011.33

Parasites_capillaria_hepatica_HC - 21308.87, 1060.91

Parasites_clonorchis_sinensis_HC - 21259.08, 1058.43

Parasites_cryptocotyle_lingua_HC - 20611.85, 1026.20

Parasites_dirofilaria_immitis_HC (dog heartworm) - 20362.91, 1013.81

Parasites_echinoparyphium_recurvatum_HC - 20960.36, 1043.55

Parasites_echinostoma_revolutum_HC - 21308.87, 1060.91

Parasites_enterobiasis (pinworms; intestinal worms which cause itching of the anal and perianal areas) - 20, 112, 120, 773, 826, 827, 835, 4152

Parasites_enterobius_vermicularis_HC - 21059.93, 1048.51

Parasites_eurytrema_pancreaticum_HC - 20960.36, 1043.55

Parasites_fasciola_hepatica_HC - 21159.50, 1053.47

Parasites_fasciola_hepatica_cercariac_HC - 21259.08, 1058.43

Parasites_fasciola_hepatica_eggs_HC - 21159.50, 1053.47

Parasites_fasciola_hepatica_miracidia_HC - 21059.93, 1048.51

Parasites_fasciola_hepatica_rediae_HC - 21159.50, 1053.47

Parasites_fasciolopsis_buskii_adult_HC - 21607.59, 1075.78

Parasites_fasciolopsis_buskil_eggs_HC - 21607.59, 1075.78

Parasites_fasciolopsis_cercariae_HC - 21607.59, 1075.78

Parasites_fasciolopsis_miracidia_HC - 21607.59, 1075.78

Parasites_fasciolopsis_rediae_HC - 21508.01, 1070.82

Parasites_filariose (worms in blood and organs of mammals, larvae passed from biting insects) - 112, 120, 332, 753

Parasites_fischoedrius_elongatus_HC - 22005.88, 1095.61

Parasites_flukes_blood - 847, 867, 329, 419, 635, 7391, 5516, 9889

Parasites_flukes_general (pancreatic, liver, and intestinal) - 6766, 6672, 6641, 6578, 2150, 2128, 2082, 2013, 2008, 2003, 2000, 1850, 945, 854, 846, 830, 763, 676, 651, 524, 435, 275, 142

Parasites_flukes_general_short_set - 524, 854, 651

Parasites_flukes_intestinal (2127/2128*) - 524, 651, 676, 844, 848, 854, 2128, 2008, 2084, 2150, 6766

Parasites_flukes_liver - 143, 275, 676, 763, 238, 6641, 6672

Parasites_flukes_lymph - 10050, 157

Parasites_flukes_pancreatic_1 - 1850, 2000, 2003, 2008, 2013, 2050, 2080, 6578

Parasites_flukes_sheep_liver - 826, 830, 834

Parasites_follicular_mange - 253, 693, 701, 774

Parasites_gastrothylax elongatus_HC - 22653.12, 1127.83

Parasites_general_1 - 4412, 2400, 2112, 1862, 1550, 800, 732, 728, 712, 688, 676, 644, 422, 128, 120

Parasites_general_2 - 10000, 3176, 1998, 1865, 1840, 880, 800, 780, 770, 740, 728, 727, 690, 665, 660, 465, 444, 440, 125, 120, 95, 80, 72, 47

Parasites_general_alternative_v - 4122, 1522, 967, 942, 854, 829, 827, 749, 741, 732, 633, 605, 604, 591, 524, 422, 411, 344, 172, 102

Parasites_general_comprehensive - 10000, 5000, 4412, 2720, 2400, 2112, 1864, 1550, 1360, 880, 854, 800, 784, 751, 732, 728, 712, 688, 651, 644, 524, 465, 442, 422, 334, 240, 152, 128, 125, 120, 112, 96, 72, 64, 20

Parasites_general_short_set - 20, 64, 72, 96, 112, 120, 152, 651, 732, 1360, 2720, 10000

Parasites_gen_custom2_TR (sweep 2000 to 2008 by 1 dwell 360) – 6578, 2000, 831, 2000, 2008, 2520, 689, 750, 880, 650, 187

Parasites_giardia - 5768, 5429, 4334, 2163, 2018, 1442, 829, 812, 721, 407, 334

Parasites_giardia_lamblia_HC - 21109.72, 1050.99

Parasites_gyrodactylus_HC -18919.09, 941.93

Parasites_haemonchus_contortus_HC - 19566.32, 974.15

Parasites_heartworms - 543, 2322, 200, 535, 1077, 799, 728

Parasites_helminthsporium (worm eggs) - 793, 969, 164, 5243

Parasites_hookworm - 6.8, 440, 2008, 6436, 5868

Parasites_leishmania_braziliensis - 787

Parasites_leishmania_braziliensis_HC - 20064.19, 998.94

Parasites_leishmania_donovani - 525, 781

Parasites_leishmania_donovani_HC - 19914.83, 991.50

Parasites_leishmania_mexicana_HC - 20014.40, 996.46

Parasites_leishmania_tropica – 791

Parasites_leishmania_tropica_HC - 20163.76, 1003.89

Parasites_loa_loa_HC - 17973.13, 894.83

Parasites_macracanthorhynchus_HC - 21906.31, 1090.65

Parasites_metagonimus Yokogawai _HC - 21906.31, 1090.65

Parasites_nematode - 771

Parasites_onchocerca_volvulus_HC (tumor) - 21906.31, 1090.65

Parasites_paragonimus_Westermanil_HC - 22503.75, 1120.40, 22254.82, 1108.00

Parasites_passalurus_ambiguus_HC - 21956.10, 1093.13, 21756.95, 1083.21

Parasites_pinworm (use Parasites, enterobiasis)

Parasites_roundworms_comp - 7159, 5897, 4412, 4152, 3212, 2720, 2322, 1372, 1113, 1077, 1054, 942, 835, 827, 826, 822, 799, 776, 773, 772, 753, 752, 749, 746, 738, 732, 728, 722, 721, 698, 688, 650, 543, 541, 535, 422, 380, 332, 240, 200, 152, 128, 120, 112, 104, 101, 20

Parasites_roundworms_general - 7159, 5897, 4412, 4152, 3212, 2720, 942, 835, 827, 772, 732, 721, 688, 650, 543, 422, 332, 240, 152, 128, 120, 112, 104, 20

Parasites_roundworms_general_short_set - 128, 152, 240, 422, 650, 688

Parasites_roundworms_flatworms_TR (use when there is chronic pain from these. 40 min each with converge 1 0.03125 or 1 0.03333) – 6187.5, 6468.8, 5050

Parasites_scabies (follicular mange which is contagious dermatitis found in many animals that is caused by mites and in which the principle activity is at the hair follicles. Use 90, 94, 98, 102, 106, 110, 253, 693 for 10 min. Scan 90 to 110 on lesser frequency intervals if needed. Also, rub skin with olive oil, let sit, then rinse with thyme tea) - 920, 1436, 2871, 5742, 90, 94, 98, 102, 106, 110, 253, 693

Parasites_schistosoma_haematobium (blood flukes) - 847, 867, 635

Parasites_schistosoma_haematobium_HC - 23549.28, 1172.45

Parasites_schistosoma_mansoni (blood fluke which can cause symptoms identical to hepatitis C) - 329, 9889

Parasites_stephanurus_dentalus (ova) - 22951.84, 1142.70

Parasites_strongyloides (threadworm, genus of roundworms) - 332, 422, 721, 732, 749, 942, 3212, 4412

Parasites_strongyloides_HC (filariform larva) - 19914.83, 991.50

Parasites_strongyloides_secondary - 380, 698, 752, 776, 722, 738, 746, 1113

Parasites_taenia (use Parasites, tapeworms)

Parasites_tapeworms (if any of these frequencies are felt strongly, also use a good herbal antiparasitic regimen plus CoQ10 in large amounts, 187*, 5522*) - 164, 187, 453, 523, 542, 623, 843, 854, 1223, 803, 1360, 3032, 5522

Parasites_tapeworms_echinococcinum (tapeworms found in dogs, wolves, cats, & rodents that can infect man, 5522*) - 164, 453, 542, 623, 5522

Parasites_tapeworms_secondary - 142, 187, 624, 662

Parasites_threadworms (use Parasites, strongyloides)

Parasites_trichinella_spiralis_HC (found in muscle) - 20138.87, 1002.66

Parasites_trichinosis - 101, 541, 822, 1054, 1372

Parasites_trichomonas_vaginalis_HC - 18968.87, 944.40

Parasites_trichuris_sp_HC (male) - 20213.55, 1006.37

Parasites_trypanosoma_brucel_HC - 21358.65, 1063.38

Parasites_trypanosoma_cruzi_HC (brain tissue) - 23051.41, 1147.66

Parasites_trypanosoma_equiperdum_HC - 22055.67, 1098.09, 22005.88, 1095.61, 21707.16, 1080.74

Parasites_trypanosoma gambiense_HC - 19715.68, 981.59

Parasites_trypanosoma_lewisi_HC (blood smear) - 21159.50, 1053.47

Parasites_trypanosoma_rhodesiense_TR - 21209.29, 1055.95
Parasites_turbatrix - 104
Parasites_urocleidus_HC - 22254.82, 1108.00

Hulda Clark zapper is indicated here.

Suggested points:
ST 25
Ren 6

Pertussis

Pertussis (whooping cough) - 526, 765, 46, 284, 9101, 697, 906
Pertussis_secondary - 880, 832, 802, 787, 776, 727, 1234, 7344

Suggested points:
Jia Ji of UB 13
LU 7

Pneumonia

Pneumococcus (use Streptococcus pneumoniae)
Pneumocystis_carnii (fungus which causes pneumonia usually developing in the immune suppressed or in infants) - 204, 340, 742
Pneumonia_1 - 10346.56, 10976.38, 5045.03, 5548.59, 5549.22, 5554.69, 5554.84, 5558.75, 5560.78, 5562.5, 6752.01, 7118.2, 7255, 7284.06, 7414.28, 7631.09, 7632.66, 7667.38, 7676.94, 8045.81, 8041.5, 10334.06, 8082.59, 8305.19, 8911.25, 9113.5, 9141.5, 9393.13, 6654.69
Pneumonia_2 - 986, 987, 988
Pneumonia_bronchial (inflammation of bronchii and lungs) - 550, 802, 880, 787, 776, 727, 452, 1474, 578
Pneumonia_general (see also Pneumonia klebsiella, Pneumonia mycoplasma, Pneumonia bronchial, Pneumonocystis carnii, Streptococcus pneumoniae. If no or slow results, try Mycoplasma General set.)
- 7660, 7344, 5000, 3702, 3672, 2688, 1862, 1550, 1238, 1234, 1200, 975, 880, 802, 787, 780, 778, 776, 774, 772, 770, 768, 766, 727, 688, 683, 660, 450, 412, 352, 20
Pneumonia_general_v - 6007, 5423, 5421, 5420, 5419, 2688, 2581, 2356, 967, 877, 838, 765, 748, 746, 568, 542, 532, 522, 520, 440
Pneumonia_mycoplasma (a contagious pneumonia of children and young adults. See also Mycoplasma General) - 688, 975, 777, 2688, 660, 709.2, 2838.5
Pneumonia_walking (use Pneumonia mycoplasma)
Pneumoniae_klebsiella (causes an acute, bacterial pneumonia) - 840, 818, 783, 779, 776, 766, 765,746, 413, 412
Pneumoniae_klebsiella_HC – 19964.61, 20860.78, 1038.60, 993.98

Suggested points:
Jia Ji of UB 13
LU 7

RSV (respiratory syncytial virus)

Respiratory_syncytial_virus - 336, 712, 278
Respiratory_syncytial_virus_HC – 18919.09, 941.93

Suggested points:
Jia Ji of UB 13
LU 7

Salmonella

Salmonella (1) - 718.2, 713.3

Salmonella (can cause intestinal inflammation and infection, and contribute to flu in children) - 1522,
718, 717, 713, 972, 664, 643

Salmonella_comp - 8656, 7771, 6787, 1634, 1522, 1244, 972, 773, 762, 754, 752, 719, 718.2, 717,
713.3, 711, 707, 693, 664, 643, 546, 420, 165, 92, 59

Salmonella_enteriditis_HC (causes intestinal infection) – 16379.95, 815.51

Salmonella_paratyphi_B - 59, 92, 643, 707, 717, 719, 752, 972, 7771, 1244, 6787, 165, 711

Salmonella_paratyphi_HC – 18321.64, 912.18Salmonella_type_B - 546, 1634

Salmonella_typhi (can cause typhoid fever) - 420, 664, 8656, 773

Salmonella_typhimurium - 693, 754, 762

Salmonella_typhimurium_HC (can cause food poisoning, nervousness, apathy) – 19168.02, 19217.81, 954.32, 956.80

Suggested points:
ST 25
Ren 12

Scabies

Scabies (use Parasites_scabies and Mange_follicular)

Parasites_scabies (follicular mange which is contagious dermatitis found in many animals that is caused by mites and in which the principle activity is at the hair follicles. Use 90, 94, 98, 102, 106, 110, 253, 693 for 10 min. Scan 90 to 110 on lesser frequency intervals if needed. Also, rub skin with olive oil, let sit, then rinse with thyme tea) - 920, 1436, 2871, 5742, 90, 94, 98, 102, 106, 110, 253, 693

Mange_follicular - 253, 693

Suggested points:
Ashi

Shingles

Herpes_zoster (chicken pox, shingles. 664*) - 3343, 2320, 2170, 1600, 1500, 1160, 914, 880, 833, 802, 787, 664, 580, 3.9
Herpes_zoster_1 (4 min each freq) - 10000, 833, 802, 3.9
Herpes_zoster_secondary - 1550, 802, 1800, 1865, 728, 2720, 2128, 5000, 464, 800, 574, 1557, 304, 20
Herpes_zoster_v - 7160, 3343, 2431, 2323, 1577, 1544, 40887, 958, 934, 787, 786, 738, 718, 716, 686, 668, 643, 576, 574, 573, 572, 563, 554, 542, 453, 446, 436, 425, 423, 411, 345, 333, 223, 134

Other: Beck Protocols are said to be effective for this condition.

Suggested points:
Du 14
Jia Ji of UB 18

Staph Infection

Staph infection_1 - 943, 727, 643, 20
Staph_and_Strep_v - 40887, 9646, 7160, 2431, 1902, 1109, 1060, 1050, 1010, 985, 958, 934, 786, 727, 718, 686, 643, 576, 563, 542, 453, 436, 423, 411, 333, 134, 128
Staphylococci_infection (see also other Staph freqs, 727*, 786*) - 960, 727, 786, 453, 678, 674, 550, 1109, 424, 943, 1050, 643, 2600, 7160, 639, 1089, 8697
Staphylococcus_aureus (can cause boils, carbuncles, abscesses, tooth infection, heart disease, and infect tumors, 786*) - 8697, 7270, 1050, 999, 943, 824.4, 787, 784, 745, 738, 728, 727, 647, 644, 555, 478, 424
Staphylococcus_aureus_HC (tooth infection, abscesses, heart disease, invades tumors) - 18819.51, 936.97, 18968.87, 944.40
Staphylococcus_coagulae_positive - 643
Staphylococcus_comp - 40887, 9646, 8697, 7270, 7160, 2600, 2431, 1902, 1109, 1089, 1060, 1050, 1010, 999, 985, 960, 958, 943, 934, 884, 882, 880, 878, 876, 824.4, 787, 786, 784, 745, 738, 728, 727, 718, 686, 678, 674, 647, 644, 643, 639, 634, 576, 563, 555, 550, 542, 478, 453, 436, 424, 423, 411, 333, 134, 128
Staphylococcus_general (728*, 786*) - 7160, 1109, 1089, 885, 884, 883, 882, 881, 880, 879, 878, 877, 876, 875, 786, 728, 674, 639, 634, 550, 453

Suggested points:
Ashi

Strep Throat

Streptococcus_infection_general (streptococcus family. Also see General antiseptic and other Strep sets, 880*) - 2000, 1266, 885, 884, 883, 882, 881, 880, 879, 878, 877, 876, 875, 848, 802, 800, 787, 784, 727

Suggested points:
ST 9
LI 4

Syphilis

Syphilis - 6600, 789, 900, 2776, 177, 650, 625, 600, 660, 658

Suggested points:
Liver 12, Bilateral

Urinary Tract Infection

Urinary_Tract_Infections (also see Bacterium_coli sets) - 2050, 880, 1550, 802, 787, 727, 465, 20, 9.39, 642, 358, 539
Bacterial_infections_general (if bacterial infection is chronic and the type is accurately diagnosed and neither frequencies nor antibiotics are effective long term, also use Parasites general and roundworms sets. Also see General antiseptic and specific types.) - 20, 465, 866, 664, 690, 727, 787, 832, 800, 880, 1550, 784
Bacterium_coli (a type of E. coli normally found in the intestines, water, milk, and soil that is the most frequent cause of urinary-tract infections and a common cause of wound infection) - 642, 358, 539
Bacterium_coli_commune_combination - 282, 333, 413, 957, 1320, 1722

Suggested points:
LIV 10, Bilateral

Warts

Warts_general (also see Papilloma and Parasites roundworms and Parasites, flukes general) - 2720, 2489, 2170, 2127, 2008, 1800, 1600, 1500, 907, 915, 874, 727, 690, 666, 660, 644, 767, 953, 495, 466, 110
Warts_1 (apply with pad at negative 24v for 5 min at a time) - 21750
Warts_papilloma (branch or stalk, use Papilloma virus)
Warts_plantar (use 915 and 918 for 15 to 30min) - 915, 918, 20, 120, 727.5, 787, 880, 2008, 2127.5
Warts_verruca (a rough surfaced, supposedly harmless, viral caused skin wart) - 495, 644, 767, 797, 877, 953, 173, 787

Suggested points:
Ashi

GEORGE LAKHOVSKY

George Lakhovky was a Russian inventor, who immigrated to France. His theory was that normal cells all resonate at certain frequencies. These frequencies are promoted by healthy diet and by resonance with normal cosmic radiation passing through the body from deep space. This will strengthen and and vitalize cells.

When these healthy frequencies are blocked or impeded, ill health would result. Pathogenic microbes inside the body resonate at different frequencies than the normal cells. This will create a dissonance between the cells and the pathogenic microbes. The process of illness is, for **Lakhovsky**, a tug of war between these two sets of frequencies.

Lakhovsky experimented with strengthening the resonance of the harmful cells, and his experimental subjects died. **Lakhovsky** experimented a lot with plants. In other experiments, he strengthened the healthy resonant frequencies of normal cells. In these cases, not only did the plants recover, but they went on to thrive.

Lakhovsky includes photos of these plants in his book, **The Secret of Life**.

Lakhovsky's device, the **Multiple Wave Oscillator**, or **MWO**, consisted of two sets of copper coils, suspended on silk threads. The patient would sit between them, and would be exposed to healthy frequencies, strengthening the functioning of normal cells. Many positive results were reported.

During World War Two, **Lakhovsky** escaped the Nazi occupation of France to the United States and ended up in New York. His machines were being experimentally evaluated by a number of hospitals at this time. However, in 1942 at the age of 73, **Lakhovsky** was killed in an automobile accident. As a result of this tragedy, this line of researched ceased.

The **MWO** was later discovered by **Bob Beck**, who stumbled upon one of the devices in the basement of a California hospital in 1963. **Beck** was an inventor of alternative health devices in his own right. He studied the **MWO** and wrote a series of articles on it for Borderlands Journal. This sparked interest in the device. A handbook was later developed.

We don't know of any good biographies of **Lakhovsky**, but his book **The Secret of Life** is very interesting. It's not new-agey in the least. We found it to be a very scientifically oriented document. It's a little far out in some respects, but it's very good.

We value **Lakhovsky**'s work in that he wants to strengthen the vitality of healthy cellular tissue. Most of the people who use frequency medicine focus on **Rife. Rife** wanted to kill the bad cells. And that's great. But to us, that's kind of a Western approach. We are TCM practitioners, so we want to have a more positive focus on promoting health. And really, couldn't it be argued that **Lakhovsky** was tonifying qi? Or moving qi and blood? We can certainly interpret his results from the standpoint of TCM.

This was our approach in the development of our method. We wanted to develop frequencies and sets of frequencies that would promote TCM-based functions and indications. We believe we have done that. The **MWO** produced numerous frequencies simultaneously, all of which would resonate with healthy bodily functions. Our devices only produce a few, but we have (we believe) developed sets of frequencies with functional harmonics, producing specifically targeted sets of desired effects. We hope they work for all of you as well as they have worked for us.

Materia Medica

of

Electroherbalism Frequencies

NOTE: As always, our frequencies are derived from the CAFL, which exists at the following link:

http://www.electroherbalism.com/Bioelectronics/FrequenciesandAnecdotes/CAFL.htm

Each frequency should be applied for a minimum of 3-5 minutes. We list our frequency sets from lower to higher. This allows us to skip over the lower frequencies straight to the higher, in cases in which patients might find the lower frequencies to be uncomfortable. All frequencies are in Hertz.

For other frequency lists, consult the various manufacturers of electroherbalism machines. Many of the manufacturers will have their own frequency lists. See also **Nenah Sylver's** excellent **Rife Handbook of Frequency Therapy.**

Astringe

Primary: 20, 40, 72, 440, 727, 880
Secondary: 125, 787, 1550,
Tertiary: 8, 28, 60, 95, 146, 250, 444, 465, 600, 625, 751, 784, 800, 1500, 1600, 1865, 10000

Bi Syndrome

Primary: 20, 727, 776, 787, 880
Secondary: 125, 240, 304, 802, 1550, 6000, 10000
Tertiary: 0.5, 1, 1.2, 1.5, 2.5, 4.9, 5.8, 6, 6.8, 9.19, 10, 40, 80, 160, 250, 300, 320, 328, 728, 766, 1500, 1800

Calm the Shen

Primary: 7.83, 6000, 10000
Secondary: 1.1, 3.5, 73, 95, 800

Clear Heat

Primary: 20, 465, 660, 727, 776, 787, 802, 832, 880, 1489, 1550, 1800, 2489, 2720, 2950, 10000
Secondary: 46.5, 141, 200, 342, 428, 467, 476, 574, 629, 664, 712, 728, 734, 745, 747, 766, 784, 875, 885, 962, 1000, 1500, 1600, 1614, 1865
Tertiary: 3.9, 116, 142, 165, 214, 222, 262, 304, 322, 339, 343, 360, 362, 366, 368, 370, 373, 383, 432, 440, 443, 446, 450, 459, 464, 480, 520, 521, 522, 528, 532, 540, 542, 552, 554, 556, 589, 590, 591, 647, 648, 650, 652, 656, 665, 685, 700, 716, 717, 718, 725, 731, 732, 733, 757, 763, 770, 778, 782, 783, 785, 800, 808, 822, 833, 843, 845, 846, 847, 848, 888,944, 1043, 1402, 1488, 1577, 1644, 1850, 1871, 2062, 2154, 3343, 3552, 3742, 4192, 5000, 5310, 5641, 8650, 8778, 14080, 34464

Cool the Blood

Primary: 9.19, 95

Drain Damp

Primary: 20, 146, 160, 320, 440, 464, 522, 727, 776, 787, 802, 880, 952, 1550, 5000
Secondary: 72, 95, 125, 444, 660, 666, 682, 690, 741, 987, 1234, 1862, 2050, 2128, 2688, 10000
Tertiary: 6.3, 9.1, 120, 148, 412, 615, 683, 688, 728, 765, 766, 975, 1500, 2008, 2250, 2600, 2720, 7344

Food Stagnation

Primary: 20, 727, 832, 880
Secondary: 72, 95, 125, 422, 444, 787, 802, 1550, 10000

Move Qi and Blood

Primary: 20, 95, 666, 727, 776, 787, 802, 880, 1550, 2720, 3000, 10000
Secondary: 1.2, 40, 80, 120, 125, 250, 304, 464, 600, 690, 728, 800, 1600, 2008, 2489, 5000, 6000
Tertiary: 3, 9.39, 9.6, 28, 160, 240, 320, 324, 465, 500, 650, 760, 1800, 2127

Nourish Blood

Primary: 20, 120, 464, 465, 727, 728, 787, 802, 880, 1550, 2720, 5000, 10000
Secondary: 40, 95, 125, 428, 660, 666, 676, 690, 760, 786, 786, 800, 800, 1488, 2008, 2128, 2489, 3176
Tertiary: 9.39, 47, 72, 424, 444, 450, 600, 664, 688, 740, 776, 776, 784, 784, 1862, 1865, 2000, 2112, 2127, 2145, 2791, 3347, 5611

Nourish Yin

Primary: 20, 95, 120, 166, 430, 444, 465, 470, 600, 620, 624, 625, 650, 660, 690, 727, 728, 776, 787, 800, 802, 840, 880, 1550, 1850, 2008, 2128, 2213, 2720, 3000, 5000, 10000
Secondary: 1.2, 7.69, 10, 28, 35, 60, 72, 100, 125, 224, 275, 440, 464, 524, 666, 784, 786, 854, 866, 1500, 1600, 1800, 1865, 2127, 2170, 2489, 5148
Tertiary: 8, 9.6, 23.2, 33, 80.9, 110, 112, 143, 190, 212, 218, 240, 241.68, 242, 246, 300, 303, 304, 304.6, 305, 317, 428, 484, 528, 680, 742.4, 760, 832, 2000, 2003, 2013, 2050, 2088.59, 2112, 2252.8, 2358, 2466.9, 2467, 3040, 3056.9, 3057, 19180.5, 23570.5

Open Orifice

Primary: 20, 802, 10000
Secondary: 7.82, 1500, 1550,

Parasites

Primary: 112, 120, 128, 152, 422, 524, 651, 688, 728, 732, 854, 2008, 4412
Secondary: 20, 72, 104, 164, 187, 240, 332, 543, 650, 676, 721, 749, 800, 826, 827, 835, 880, 942, 991.50, 1053.47, 1090.65, 1360, 2000, 2720, 3212, 4152, 6578, 10000, 21159.50, 21607.59, 21906.31
Tertiary: 64, 96, 101, 102, 125, 142, 200, 253, 275, 329, 334, 380, 440, 442, 453, 465, 535, 541, 542, 623, 635, 644, 693, 698, 712, 722, 738, 746, 751, 752, 753, 763, 772, 773, 776, 799, 822, 829, 830, 847, 867, 974.15, 1011.33, 1043.55, 1048.51, 1054, 1058.43, 1060.91, 1095.61, 1108.00, 1113, 1372, 1550, 1850, 2003, 2013, 2112, 2128, 2150, 2322, 2400, 5522, 5897, 6641, 6672, 6766, 7159, 9889, 19566.32, 19914.83, 20313.12, 20960.36, 21059.93, 21259.08, 21308.87, 22005.88, 22254.82

Release the Exterior

Primary: 440, 727, 776, 787, 802, 880, 1550, 10000
Secondary: 20, 72, 125, 146, 522, 683, 688, 766, 1234, 2489, 5000, 7344
Tertiary: 7.83, 27.57, 33, 47.5, 304, 333, 444, 465, 600, 650, 660, 720, 728, 746, 768, 800, 1800, 3176

Resolve Phlegm

Primary: 20, 95, 125, 304, 465, 666, 690, 727, 728, 776, 784, 787, 800, 802, 880, 1550, 1552, 2008, 2127, 2128, 2182, 2184, 2189, 2217, 2720, 3672, 10000
Secondary: 10, 60, 72, 120, 422, 428, 444, 450, 464, 478, 524, 543, 641, 650, 660, 664, 676, 760, 766, 778, 822, 832, 854, 857, 1050, 1234, 1384, 1488, 1744, 1865, 2000, 2005, 2030, 2048, 2050, 2084, 2100, 2104, 2112, 2116, 2120, 2145, 2160, 2170, 2180, 2489, 2876, 2950, 3040, 3176, 3524, 3713, 5000, 10025, 11780, 17034, 21275
Tertiary: 6.8, 7.5, 45, 66.5, 80, 96, 100, 127, 178, 190, 222, 249, 262, 263.11, 267, 333, 334, 414, 418, 440, 442, 466, 475, 482, 488, 495, 500, 523, 552, 600, 647, 656, 665, 731, 732, 781, 785, 852, 866, 979, 982, 1000, 1340, 1489, 1566.4, 1582, 1600, 1604, 1675, 1840, 1862, 1998, 2012, 2016, 2093, 2127.5, 2136, 2144, 2152, 2385, 2452, 2521, 2586, 2655, 2663, 2787.5, 2790, 3000, 3324, 5013, 5013.5, 5020, 5122, 5278.3, 5318.8, 5388.5, 5575, 6024, 6384, 6687.3, 7037.5, 7356, 7760, 8020, 8368.2, 8610, 8836.9, 9999, 10026, 10027, 11430

Smooth Liver Qi

Primary: 26, 727, 787, 880, 10000
Secondary: 1.1, 3.5, 7.83, 73, 465, 800, 802, 1550, 6000

Spleen Qi

Primary: 20, 72, 95, 125, 440, 465, 727, 787, 802, 832, 880, 1550, 5000, 10000
Secondary: 4.9, 120, 190, 444, 664, 1552, 1865
Tertiary: 2, 3, 10, 422, 424, 447, 600, 648, 660, 786, 2127

Stop Cough

Primary: 20, 146, 727, 776, 787, 1234,
Secondary: 0.5, 7.7, 72, 95, 125, 432, 440, 444, 514, 522, 524, 525, 530, 683, 720, 728, 766, 1500, 1550, 3702, 7344

Subdue Wind

Primary: 1.2, 7.83, 10, 20, 72, 125, 727, 787, 880, 10000
Secondary: 4, 4.9, 5.8, 6, 6.3, 9.19, 9.39, 9.6, 60, 95, 470, 522, 600, 650, 802, 813, 1865, 6000

Summer Heat

Primary: 20, 440, 880, 10000

Tonify Qi

Primary: 10, 20, 40, 72, 80, 95, 120, 125, 428, 440, 444, 450, 464, 465, 600, 625, 650, 660, 666, 676, 690, 727, 728, 776, 787, 800, 802, 880, 1500, 1550, 1600, 1865, 2008, 2489, 2720, 5000, 10000
Secondary: 1.2, 7.83, 8, 9.39, 60, 73, 100, 160, 220, 240, 250, 304, 400, 422, 500, 622, 664, 688, 712, 727.5, 740, 760, 766, 784, 786, 832, 1234, 1488, 1552, 1560, 1570, 1800, 1850, 1862, 2000, 2112, 2127, 2128, 2250, 3000, 3176, 7344
Tertiary: 1, 2, 3.9, 4, 7, 14, 30, 47, 128, 146, 162, 424, 432, 568, 683, 700, 730, 732, 804, 1000, 1840, 1998, 2093, 2127.5, 2145, 2180, 3040, 3500, 3672, 40000

Tonify Yang

Primary: 72, 95, 125, 440, 465, 600, 625, 666, 690, 20 727, 787, 802, 880, 1550, 2008, 2127, 2720, 5500, 10000
Secondary: 9.39, 40, 73, 100, 120, 146, 444, 522, 650, 660, 728, 776, 800, 1234, 2050, 2112, 1500, 2250
Tertiary: 2, 3.9, 10, 80, 160, 248, 250, 410, 424, 664, 712, 746, 751, 768, 1000, 1600, 1865, 2128, 2400, 2489, 3000, 7344, 9999

Wei Qi/Vital Qi

Primary: 20, 120, 428, 465, 676, 727, 728, 760, 776, 786, 787, 800, 802, 832, 880, 1550, 2720, 5000, 10000
Secondary: 146, 444, 450, 522, 660, 666, 690, 1488, 1500, 1600, 1800, 2008, 2128, 2489, 3176
Tertiary: 40.5, 95, 125, 304, 333, 422, 440, 500, 600, 688, 732, 740, 766, 784, 1552, 1862, 1865, 2000, 2112, 3040, 40000

Materia Medica

Of

Harmonic Frequencies

Based upon

TCM Herbal Formulas

NOTE: As always, our frequencies are derived from the CAFL, which exists at the following link:

http://www.electroherbalism.com/Bioelectronics/FrequenciesandAnecd otes/CAFL.htm

Each frequency should be applied for a minimum of 3-5 minutes. We list our frequency sets from lower to higher. This allows us to skip over the lower frequencies straight to the higher, in cases in which patients might find the lower frequencies to be uncomfortable. All frequencies are in Hertz.

For other frequency lists, consult the various manufacturers of electroherbalism machines. Many of the manufacturers will have their own frequency lists. See also **Nenah Sylver's** excellent **Rife Handbook of Frequency Therapy.**

Bai He Gu Jin Tang

Primary: 20, 95, 465, 650, 660, 690, 727, 728, 776, 784, 787, 800, 802, 832, 880, 1550, 1865, 2008, 2128, 2489, 2720, 5000, 10000

Secondary: 10, 20, 60, 72, 110, 125, 166, 304, 428, 428, 430, 430, 440, 444, 450, 464, 470, 524, 600, 620, 624, 625, 664, 747, 760, 766, 778, 822, 840, 854, 866, 1000, 1488, 1489, 1500, 1552, 1600, 1800, 1850, 2000, 2050, 2112, 2127, 2170, 2182, 2184, 2189, 2213, 2217, 2950, 3000, 3040, 3672

Tertiary: 1.2, 7.69, 28, 35, 46.5, 141, 190, 200, 222, 224, 262, 275, 342, 422, 467, 476, 478, 528, 543, 552, 574, 629, 629, 641, 647, 656, 665, 676, 712, 731, 732, 734, 785, 786, 857, 875, 885, 1050, 1234, 1384, 1614, 1744, 2005, 2005, 2030, 2048, 2084, 2100, 2104, 2116, 2120, 2160, 2180, 2876, 3176, 3524, 3713, 5148, 10025, 11780, 12145, 17034, 21275

Suggested Points:
UB 13
DU 14

Bai Hu Tang

Primary: 20, 465, 660, 727, 728, 776, 787, 802, 880, 1550, 1800, 2489, 2720, 10000

Secondary: 95, 120, 166, 428, 430, 440, 444, 464, 470, 600, 620, 624, 625, 650, 690, 784, 800, 832, 840, 1489, 1500, 1600, 1850, 1865, 2008, 2128, 2213, 2950, 3000, 5000

Tertiary: 1.2, 7.69, 10, 28, 35, 46.5, 60, 72, 100, 125, 141, 200, 224, 275, 304, 342, 467, 476, 524, 528, 574, 629, 664, 666, 712, 734, 745, 747, 766, 786, 854, 866, 875, 885, 962, 1000, 1614, 2127, 2170, 5148

Suggested Points:
Du 14
Jia Ji of UB 23

Bai Tou Weng Tang

Primary: 20, 146, 160, 320, 440, 464, 522, 727, 776, 787, 802, 880, 952, 1550, 5000, 10000

Secondary: 9.19, 95, 304, 465, 660, 728, 766, 832, 1489, 1500, 1800, 2489, 2720, 2950

Tertiary: 46.5, 125, 141, 200, 240, 342, 428, 467, 476, 574, 629, 664, 712, 734, 745, 747, 784, 875, 885, 962, 1000, 1600, 1614, 1865, 6000

Suggested Points:
Du 14
Jia Ji of UB 17

Ban Xia Bai Zhu Tian Ma Tang

Primary: 1.2, 7.83, 20, 95, 125, 465, 600, 650, 660, 727, 728, 776, 787, 800, 802, 880, 1550, 1600, 1800, 1865, 2489, 2720, 3000, 5000, 6000, 10000

Secondary: 9.39, 9.6, 10, 60, 72, 120, 166, 304, 428, 430, 440, 444, 464, 470, 522, 620, 624, 625, 666, 690, 784, 832, 840, 1489, 1500, 1850, 2008, 2127, 2128, 2213, 2950

Tertiary: 1.1, 3.5, 4, 4.9, 5.8, 6, 6.3, 7.69, 9.19, 26, 28, 35, 40, 46.5, 73, 80, 100, 141, 200, 224, 240, 250, 275, 342, 467, 476, 524, 528, 574, 629, 664, 712, 734, 745, 747, 760, 766, 786, 813, 866, 875, 885, 962, 1000, 1614, 2170, 5148

Suggested points:
Du 14
Jia Ji of UB 18

Ban Xia Hou Pu Tang

Primary: 20, 125, 465, 660, 727, 728, 776, 784, 787, 800, 802, 832, 880, 1234, 1550, 2489, 2720, 2950, 10000

Secondary: 26, 72, 95, 146, 304, 428, 432, 440, 444, 450, 464, 522, 524, 650, 664, 666, 690, 757, 766, 778, 822, 1000, 1488, 1489, 1500, 1552, 1600, 1800, 1865, 2008, 2127, 2128, 2182, 2184, 2189, 2217, 3672, 5000

Tertiary: 0.5, 1.1, 3.5, 7.7, 7.83, 10, 46.5, 60, 73, 120, 141, 200, 222, 262, 342, 422, 467, 476, 478, 514, 525, 530, 543, 552, 574, 629, 641, 647, 656, 665, 676, 683, 712, 720, 731, 732, 734, 745, 760, 766, 785, 854, 857, 875, 885, 962, 1050, 1384, 1614, 1744, 2000, 2005, 2030, 2048, 2050, 2084, 2100, 2104, 2112, 2116, 2120, 2145, 2160, 2170, 2180, 2876, 3040, 3176, 3524, 3702, 3713, 6000, 7344, 10025, 11780, 17034, 21275

Suggested Points:
Jia Ji of UB 17
Jia Ji of UB 20

Ban Xia Xie Xin Tang

Primary: 20, 72, 95, 125, 727, 787, 802, 832, 880, 1550

Secondary: 422, 440, 444, 465, 5000, 10000

Tertiary: 4.9, 100, 120, 190, 664, 1865

Suggested points:
SP 6
ST 36

Bao He Wan

Primary: 20, 72, 95, 120, 125, 304, 444, 465, 660, 664, 666, 727, 728, 776, 787, 800, 802, 832, 880, 1550, 1865, 2489, 2720, 5000, 10000

Secondary: 10, 80, 190, 428, 440, 450, 464, 600, 650, 690, 760, 766, 778, 784, 822, 1000, 1488, 1489, 1552, 1600, 1800, 2008, 2127, 2128, 2182, 2184, 2189, 2217, 2950, 3000, 3672

Tertiary: 1.2, 3, 4.9, 40, 46.5, 60, 141, 200, 222, 250, 262, 342, 467, 476, 478, 500, 524, 543, 552, 574, 629, 641, 647, 648, 656, 665, 676, 712, 731, 732, 734, 745, 747, 785, 854, 857, 875, 885, 962, 1050, 1234, 1384, 1500, 1614, 1744, 2000, 2005, 2030, 2048, 2050, 2084, 2100, 2104, 2112, 2120, 2145, 2160, 2170, 2180, 2876, 3040, 3176, 3524, 3713, 6000, 10025, 11780, 17034, 21275

Suggested points:
Du 14
Jia Ji of UB 20

Ba Zheng San

Primary: 20, 125, 440, 465, 660, 727, 776, 787, 802, 832, 880, 1550, 5000, 10000

Secondary: 4.9, 72, 95, 120, 146, 160, 304, 320, 444, 464, 476, 522, 664, 728, 766, 952, 1489, 1500, 1800, 1865, 2489, 2720, 2950

Tertiary: 10, 46.5, 141, 190, 200, 240, 342, 428, 574, 629, 648, 666, 682, 690, 712, 734, 741, 745, 747, 784, 875, 885, 962, 987, 1000, 1234, 1552, 1600, 1614, 1862, 2050, 2128, 2688, 6000

Suggested Points:
Du 14
Jia Ji of UB 20

Ba Zhen Tang

Primary: 40, 72, 80, 95, 120, 20 125, 428, 440, 444, 464, 465, 600, 660, 664, 666, 690, 727, 728, 776, 786, 787, 800, 802, 880, 1550, 1865, 1865, 2008, 2489, 2720, 5000, 10000

Secondary: 1.2, 9.39, 10, 160, 240, 250, 304, 422, 424, 450, 500, 625, 650, 676, 688, 740, 784, 1488, 1500, 1552, 1600, 1800, 1862, 1862, 2000, 2112, 2127, 2128, 3000, 3176

Tertiary: 2, 3, 4.9, 7.83, 8, 47, 60, 73, 100, 190, 220, 400, 622, 712, 727.5, 766, 1234, 1560, 1570, 1850, 2145, 2250, 6000, 7344

Suggested Points:
Jia Ji of UB 17
Jia Ji of UB 19

Bu Yang Huan Wu Tang

Primary: 20, 40, 80, 95, 120, 125, 464, 600, 666, 690, 727, 728, 776, 787, 800, 802, 880, 1550, 1600, 2008, 2489, 2720, 3000, 5000, 10000

Secondary: 1.2, 9.39, 10, 72, 160, 240, 250, 304, 428, 440, 444, 450, 465, 500, 625, 650, 660, 676, 760, 1500, 1800, 1865, 2127

Tertiary: 7.83, 8, 60, 73, 100, 220, 400, 422, 622, 664, 688, 712, 727.5, 740, 766, 784, 786, 832, 1234, 1488, 1552, 1560, 1570, 1850, 1862, 2000, 2112, 2128, 2250, 3176, 6000, 7344

Suggested Points:
Jia Ji of UB 17
Jia Ji of UB 18

Bu Zhong Yi Qi Tang

Primary: 10, 20, 40, 72, 95, 120, 125, 440, 444, 465, 600, 625, 650, 660, 664, 666, 690, 727, 728, 776, 787, 800, 802, 832, 880, 1500, 1550, 1865, 2008, 2127, 2720, 5000, 10000

Secondary: 2, 9.39, 73, 80, 100, 146, 160, 250, 422, 424, 428, 450, 464, 676, 712, 786, 1234, 1552, 1600, 2112, 2128, 2250, 2489, 3000, 5500, 7344

Tertiary: 1.2, 3.9, 4.9, 7.83, 8, 60, 190, 220, 240, 304, 400, 500, 522, 622, 688, 727.5, 740, 760, 766, 784, 1000, 1488, 1560, 1570, 1800, 1850, 1862, 2000, 2050, 3176

Suggested Points:
Jia Ji of UB 20
Du 4

Cang Er Zhi San

Primary: 20, 125, 304, 440, 465, 660, 727, 728, 766, 776, 784, 787, 800, 802, 832, 880, 1550, 2489, 2720, 2950, 3672, 5000, 10000

Secondary: 72, 95, 428, 444, 450, 464, 522, 650, 664, 666, 690, 757, 778, 822, 1000, 1234, 1488, 1489, 1552, 1600, 1800, 1865, 2008, 2127, 2128, 2182, 2184, 2189, 2217, 3176

Tertiary: 10, 46.5, 60, 120, 141, 146, 200, 222, 262, 333, 342, 422, 467, 476, 478, 524, 543, 552, 574, 600, 629, 641, 647, 656, 665, 676, 683, 688, 712, 731, 732, 734, 745, 760, 785, 854, 857, 875, 885, 962, 1050, 1384, 1500, 1614, 1744, 2000, 2005, 2030, 2048, 2050, 2084, 2100, 2104, 2112, 2116, 2120, 2145, 2160, 2170, 2180, 2876, 3040, 3524, 3713, 7344, 10025, 11780, 17034, 21275

Suggested points:
Du 14
Jia Ji of UB 20

Chai Ge Jie Ji Tang

Primary: 20, 727, 766, 776, 787, 802, 880, 1550, 1800, 2489, 10000

Secondary: 125, 304, 440, 465, 522, 660, 728, 832, 1489, 1500, 2720, 2950, 5000

Tertiary: 46.5, 72, 141, 146, 200, 240, 342, 428, 467, 476, 574, 629, 650, 664, 683, 688, 712, 734, 745, 747, 784, 800, 885, 962, 1000, 1234, 1600, 1614, 1865, 6000, 7344

Suggested points:
Du 14
Jia Ji of UB 18

Chai Hu Shu Gan San

Primary: 727, 787, 802, 880, 1550, 10000

Secondary: 465, 666, 776, 800, 2720, 3000, 6000

Tertiary: 1.1, 1.2, 3.5, 7.83, 20, 26, 40, 73, 80, 95, 120, 125, 250, 304, 464, 600, 690, 728, 1600, 2489, 5000, 2008, 2489

Suggested points:
Du 14
Jia Ji of UB 18

Chuan Xiong Cha Tiao San

Primary: 20, 727, 776, 787, 802, 880, 1550, 10000

Secondary: 95, 125, 304, 440, 600, 666, 728, 800, 2489, 2720, 3000, 5000

Tertiary: 1.2, 40, 72, 80, 120, 146, 250, 464, 465, 522, 650, 683, 688, 690, 766, 1234, 1600, 1800, 2008, 6000, 7344

Suggested points:
Du 14
Jia Ji of UB 18

Da Bu Yin Wan

Primary: 20, 465, 660, 727, 728, 776, 787, 802, 880, 1550, 1800, 2489, 2720, 10000

Secondary: 95, 120, 166, 428, 430, 440, 444, 464, 470, 600, 620, 624, 625, 650, 690, 784, 800, 832, 840, 1489, 1500, 1600, 1850, 1865, 2008, 2128, 2213, 2950, 3000, 5000

Tertiary: 1.2, 7.69, 10, 28, 35, 46.5, 60, 72, 100, 125, 141, 200, 224, 275, 304, 342, 467, 476, 524, 528, 574, 629, 664, 666, 712, 734, 745, 747, 766, 786, 854, 866, 885, 962, 1000, 1614, 2127, 2170, 5148

Suggested points:
Du 14
Jia Ji of UB 23

Da Chai Hu Tang

Primary: 20, 727, 776, 787, 802, 880, 1550, 2489, 10000

Secondary: 440, 465, 476, 522, 660, 728, 766, 832, 1489, 1800, 2720, 2950, 5000

Tertiary: 46.5, 72, 125, 141, 146, 200, 304, 342, 428, 574, 629, 650, 664, 683, 688, 712, 734, 745, 747, 784, 800, 875, 885, 962, 1000, 1234, 1500, 1600, 1614, 1865, 7344

Suggested points:
Du 14
Jia Ji of UB 13

Da Cheng Qi Tang

Primary: 20, 727, 776, 787, 802, 880, 1550, 2489, 2720, 10000

Secondary: 95, 304, 464, 465, 660, 666, 728, 800, 832, 1489, 1600, 1800, 2950, 3000, 5000

Tertiary: 1.2, 40, 46.5, 80, 120, 125, 141, 200, 250, 342, 428, 467, 476, 574, 600, 629, 650, 664, 690, 712, 734, 745, 747, 766, 784, 875, 885, 962, 1000, 1500, 1614, 1865, 2008, 6000

Suggested points:
ST 25 bilateral

Da Jian Zhong Tang

Primary: 20, 72, 95, 120, 125, 465, 727, 728, 787, 802, 880, 1550, 2008, 2720, 5000, 10000

Secondary: 112, 128, 152, 240, 422, 440, 524, 600, 650, 651, 666, 688, 732, 776, 800, 832 854, 3000, 4412

Tertiary: 1.2, 3, 4.9, 40, 80, 104, 164, 187, 190, 250, 304, 332, 444, 464, 543, 664, 676, 690, 721, 749, 826, 827, 835, 942, 991.50, 1053.47, 1090.65, 1360, 1552, 1600, 1865, 2000, 2127, 2489, 3212, 4152, 6000, 6578, 21159.50, 21607.59, 21906.31

Suggested Points:
Jia Ji of UB 18
Jia Ji of UB 20

Dang Gui Bu Xue Tang

Primary: 20, 95, 120, 125, 465, 727, 786, 787, 802, 880, 1550, 5000, 10000

Secondary: 72, 440, 444, 464, 660, 664, 800, 832, 1865, 2720

Tertiary: 4.9, 40, 190, 424, 428, 600, 666, 676, 690, 728, 760, 776, 784, 1488, 1552, 2008, 2127, 2128, 2489, 3176

Suggested points:
Jia Ji of UB 17
Jia Ji of UB 20

Dang Gui Liu Huang Tang

Primary: 10, 20, 40, 72, 95, 110, 120, 125, 428, 440, 444, 450, 464, 465, 600, 625, 650, 660, 664, 666, 676, 690, 727, 728, 760, 776, 784, 786, 787, 800, 802, 832, 880, 1488, 1500, 1550, 1600, 1800, 1865, 2008, 2127, 2128, 2489, 2720, 3000, 5000, 10000

Secondary: 1.2, 8, 9.39, 60, 80, 166, 240, 304, 430, 470, 620, 624, 688, 712, 740, 757, 766, 840, 1000, 1489, 1850, 1862, 2000, 2112, 2213, 2950, 3176

Tertiary: 3.9, 7.69, 7.83, 28, 35, 46.5, 47, 73, 141, 160, 200, 220, 224, 250, 275, 342, 400, 422, 424, 432, 467, 476, 500, 524, 528, 574, 622, 629, 700, 727.5, 732, 734, 745, 854, 866, 875, 885, 962, 1234, 1552, 1560, 1570, 1614, 1850, 2145, 2170, 2250, 3040, 5148, 7344

Suggested points:
Du 14
Jia Ji of UB 23

Dao Chi San

Primary: 1.2, 10, 20, 72, 95, 120, 125, 304, 625, 660, 727, 728, 776, 787, 802, 880, 1500, 1550, 1600, 1800, 2170, 2489, 2720, 10000

Secondary: 2.5, 3, 3.59, 7.83, 110, 166, 428, 430, 440, 444, 464, 465, 470, 600, 620, 624, 650, 690, 784, 800, 832, 840, 1489, 1850, 1865, 2008, 2128, 2213, 2950, 3000, 5000, 6000

Tertiary: 7.69, 28, 35, 46.5, 60, 141, 200, 224, 275, 342, 465, 467, 476, 524, 528, 574, 629, 664, 666, 712, 734, 745, 747, 766, 786, 854, 866, 875, 885, 962, 1000, 1614, 2127, 5148

Suggested points:
Du 14

Jia Ji of UB 15

Ding Chuan Tang

Primary: 20, 72, 95, 125, 146, 440, 444, 727, 728, 766, 776, 787, 802,880, 1234, 1550, 10000

Secondary: 304, 465, 522, 524, 650, 660, 666, 683, 690, 720, 784, 800, 1552, 2008, 2127, 2128, 2182, 2184, 2189, 2217, 2489, 2720, 3176, 3672, 5000, 7344

Tertiary: 0.5, 7.7, 10, 60, 120, 333, 422, 428, 450, 464, 478, 514, 525, 530, 543, 600, 641, 664, 676, 688, 760, 778, 822, 832, 854, 857, 1050, 1384, 1488, 1500, 1744, 1865, 2000, 2005, 2030, 2048, 2050, 2084, 2100, 2104, 2112, 2116, 2120, 2145, 2160, 2170, 2180, 2876, 2950, 3040, 3524, 3702, 3713, 10025, 11780, 17034, 21275

Suggested points:
Du 14
Jia Ji of UB 13

Du Huo Ji Sheng Tang

Primary: 1.2, 10, 40, 72, 240, 304 440, 676, 760, 776, 784, 1500, 1550, 1600, 1800, 1850, 1865, 2008, 2127, 2128, 2489, 2720, 3000, 5000, 10000

Secondary: 8, 9.39, 60, 80, 100, 160, 166, 250, 430, 450, 470, 620, 624, 664, 688, 740, 766, 832, 840, 1488, 1862, 2000, 2112, 2213, 3176

Tertiary: 1, 7.69, 7.83, 28, 35, 47, 73, 220, 224, 275, 300, 400, 422, 424, 500, 524, 622, 712, 727.5, 854, 866, 1234, 1552, 1560, 1570, 2145, 2170, 2250, 3040, 5148, 6000, 7344

Suggested points:
Jia Ji of UB 17
Jia Ji of UB 23

Du Qi Wan

Primary: 20, 95, 120, 444, 465, 600, 625, 650, 660, 690, 727, 728, 776, 787, 800, 802, 880, 1234, 1550, 1850, 2008, 2128, 2720, 3000, 5000, 7344, 10000

Secondary: 1.2, 8, 10, 60, 72, 100, 125, 166, 240, 304, 428, 430, 440, 464, 470, 620, 624, 666, 760, 784, 786, 832, 840, 1500, 1600, 1800, 1865, 2000, 2112, 2127, 2213, 2489, 3672, 3702, 7760

Tertiary: 7.69, 7.83, 9.39, 28, 35, 40, 73, 80, 160, 220, 224, 250, 275, 400, 422, 465, 500, 524, 622, 664, 676, 688, 712, 727.5, 740, 766, 854, 866, 1488, 1552, 1560, 1570, 1862, 2170, 2250, 3040, 3176, 5148

Suggested points:
Jia Ji of UB 23
Jia Ji of UB 24

Er Chen Tang

Primary: 20, 72, 95, 120, 125, 304, 440, 444, 464, 465, 660, 666, 690, 727, 728, 776, 787, 800, 802, 832, 880, 1550, 1552, 2008, 2127, 2128, 2720, 5000, 10000

Secondary: 10, 80, 146, 160, 190, 320, 422, 522, 600, 650, 664, 760, 766, 784, 952, 1234, 1600, 1862, 1865, 2050, 2182, 2184, 2189, 2217, 2489, 3000, 3672

Tertiary: 1.2, 3, 4.9, 40, 60, 250, 428, 450, 478, 500, 524, 543, 641, 676, 682, 741, 778, 822, 854, 857, 987, 1050, 1384, 1488, 1744, 2000, 2005, 2030, 2048, 2084, 2100, 2104, 2112, 2116, 2120, 2145, 2160, 2170, 2180, 2688, 2876, 2950, 3040, 3176, 3524, 3713, 6000, 10025, 11780, 17034, 21275

Suggested Points:
Jia Ji of UB 13
Jia Ji of UB 20

Er Miao San

Primary: 20, 660, 727, 776, 787, 802, 880, 1550, 10000

Secondary: 146, 160, 320, 440, 464, 465, 522, 728, 766, 832, 952, 1489, 1500, 1800, 2489, 2720, 2950, 5000

Tertiary: 46.5, 72, 95, 125, 141, 200, 342, 428, 444, 467, 476, 574, 629, 664, 666, 682, 690, 712, 734, 741, 745, 747, 784, 875, 885, 962, 987, 1000, 1234, 1600, 1614, 1862, 1865, 2050, 2128, 2688

Suggested Points:
Du 14
Jia Ji of UB 20

Er Xian Tang

Primary: 20, 95, 120, 125, 440, 444, 465, 600, 625, 650, 660, 666, 690, 727, 728, 776, 787, 800, 802, 880, 1550, 1600, 2008, 2127, 2489, 2720, 3000, 5000, 10000

Secondary: 1.2, 9.39, 10, 28, 40, 72, 80, 100, 166, 250, 304, 430, 464, 470, 620, 624, 840, 1500, 1800, 1850, 1865, 2050, 2112, 2128, 2213, 5500

Tertiary: 7.69, 9.6, 35, 60, 73, 146, 160, 224, 240, 275, 522, 524, 760, 784, 786, 854, 866, 1234, 2170, 2250, 5148, 6000

Suggested points:
Jia Ji of UB 23
Du 4

Er Zhi Wan

Primary: 20, 95, 120, 464, 465, 660, 690, 727, 728, 776, 786, 787, 800, 802, 880, 1550, 2008, 2128, 2720, 5000, 10000

Secondary: 26, 72, 125, 166, 428, 430, 444, 470, 600, 620, 624, 625, 650, 666, 760, 784, 840, 1850, 1865, 2127, 2213, 2489, 3000

Tertiary: 1.1, 1.2, 3.5, 7.69, 7.83, 10, 28, 35, 60, 73, 100, 224, 275, 440, 524, 676, 854, 866, 1488, 1500, 1600, 1800, 2000, 2112, 2170, 3176, 5148, 6000

Suggested points:
Jia Ji of UB 18
Jia Ji of UB 23

Fu Yuan Huo Xue Tang

Primary: 727, 787, 802, 880, 1550, 10000

Secondary: 20, 26, 95, 465, 666, 776, 800, 2720, 3000, 6000

Tertiary: 1.1, 3.5, 7.83, 40, 73, 80, 120, 125, 250, 304, 464, 600, 690, 728, 1600, 2008, 2489, 5000

Suggested points:
Jia Ji of UB 17
Jia Ji of UB 18

Gan Mai Da Zao Tang

Primary: 10, 20, 72, 95, 120, 125, 440, 444, 464, 465, 600, 625, 650, 660, 666, 690, 727, 728, 776, 787, 800, 802, 880, 1500, 1550, 1600, 1850, 1865, 2008, 2128, 2213, 2489, 2720, 3000, 5000, 10000

Secondary: 1.2, 7.83, 8, 26, 40, 60, 73, 80, 100, 166, 240, 304, 428, 430, 450, 470, 620, 624, 676, 760, 784, 786, 832, 840, 1800, 2000, 2127, 2250

Tertiary: 1.1, 3.5, 7.69, 9.39, 28, 35, 160, 220, 224, 250, 275, 400, 422, 500, 622, 664, 524, 688, 740, 766, 854, 866, 1234, 1488, 1552, 1560, 1570, 1862, 2112, 2170, 3040, 3176, 5148, 6000, 7344

Suggested points:
Jia Ji of UB 18
Jia ji of UB 23

Gan Mao Ling

Primary: 20, 727, 776, 787, 802, 880, 1550, 2489, 10000

Secondary: 440, 465, 476, 522, 660, 728, 766, 832, 1489, 1800, 2720, 2950, 5000

Tertiary: 46.5, 72, 125, 141, 146, 200, 304, 342, 428, 574, 629, 650, 664, 683, 688, 712, 734, 745, 747, 784, 800, 885, 962, 1000, 1234, 1500, 1600, 1614, 1865, 7344,

Suggested points:
Du 14
Jia Ji of UB 13

Ge Gen Huang Lian Huang Qin Tang

Primary: 20, 146, 440, 522 727, 776, 787, 802, 880, 1550, 5000, 10000

Secondary: 72, 125, 160, 320, 444, 464, 660, 683, 688, 766 952, 1234, 7344

Tertiary: 95, 666, 682, 690, 728, 741, 987, 1862, 2050, 2128, 2489, 2688

Suggested points
DU 14
Jia Ji of UB 20

Ge Gen Tang

Primary: 20, 125, 440, 727, 728, 776, 787, 802, 880, 1550, 5000, 10000

Secondary: 1.2, 72, 304, 444, 465, 600, 620, 624, 625, 650, 660, 800, 840, 1500, 1800, 1850, 2008, 2128, 2213, 2489, 2720, 3000

Tertiary: 7.69, 10, 28, 33, 35, 60, 95, 100, 120, 146, 166, 224, 240, 275, 300, 430, 464, 470, 522, 524, 666, 683, 688, 690, 766, 784, 786, 854, 866, 1234, 1600, 1865, 2127, 2170, 5148, 6000, 7344

Suggested points:
DU 14
Jia Ji of UB 23

Ge Xia Zhu Yu Tang

Primary: 20, 50, 95, 120, 464, 465, 666, 727, 728, 776, 787, 800, 802, 880, 1550, 2720, 10000

Secondary: 26, 40, 125, 600, 690, 760, 786, 2008, 2489, 3000, 6000

Tertiary: 1.1, 1.2, 3.5, 7.83, 9.39, 73, 80, 250, 304, 424, 428, 660, 676, 784, 1488, 1600, 2127, 2128, 2128, 3176

Suggested points:
Jia Ji of UB 17
Jia Ji of UB 18

Gui Pi Tang

Primary: 20, 72, 95, 120, 125, 440, 444, 464, 465, 600, 660, 690, 727, 728, 776, 786, 786, 787, 800, 802, 880, 1550, 1865, 2008, 2128, 2720, 5000, 10000

Secondary: 10, 110, 166, 190, 428, 430, 470, 620, 624, 625, 650, 664, 666, 760, 832, 840, 1850, 2127, 2213, 2489, 3000

Tertiary: 1.2, 4.9, 7.69, 28, 35, 40, 60, 224, 275, 424, 524, 676, 854, 866, 1488, 1500, 1552, 1600, 1800, 2000, 2112, 2170, 3176, 5148

Suggested points:
Jia Ji of SP 15
Jia Ji of SP 20

Gui Zhi Shao Yao Zhi Mu Tang

Primary: 20, 95, 125, 160, 320, 464, 666, 727, 776, 787, 802, 880, 1550, 5000, 10000

Secondary: 1.2, 40, 80, 120, 146, 240, 250, 304, 440, 522, 690, 728, 952, 2008, 2720, 3000, 6000

Tertiary: 72, 444, 600, 660, 682, 741, 800, 987, 1234, 1500, 1600, 1800, 1862, 2050, 2128, 2489, 2688

Suggested Points:
Jia Ji of UB 18
Jia Ji of UB 20

Gui Zhi Tang

Primary: 20, 727, 776, 787, 802, 880, 1550, 10000

Secondary: 95, 125, 304, 440, 600, 666, 728, 800, 2489, 2720, 3000, 5000

Tertiary: 1.2, 40, 72, 80, 120, 146, 250, 464, 465, 522, 650, 683, 688, 690, 766, 1234, 1600, 1800, 2008, 6000, 7344

Suggested points:
Du 14
Jia Ji of UB 13

Gui Zi Fu Ling Wan

Primary: 20, 95, 125, 304, 666, 690, 727, 728, 776, 787, 800, 802, 880, 1550, 2008, 2720, 10000

Secondary: 80, 120, 464, 465, 600, 650, 760, 784, 1552, 1600, 2127, 2128, 2182, 2184, 2189, 2217, 2489, 3000, 3672, 5000

Tertiary: 1.2, 10, 40, 60, 72, 250, 422, 428, 444, 450, 478, 500, 524, 543, 641, 660, 664, 676, 766, 778, 822, 832, 854, 857, 1050, 1234, 1384, 1488, 1744, 1865, 2000, 2005, 2030, 2048, 2050, 2084, 2100, 2104, 2112, 2116, 2120, 2145, 2160, 2170, 2180, 2876, 2950, 3040, 3176, 3524, 3713, 6000, 10025, 11780, 17034, 21275

Suggested points:
Jia Ji of UB 18
Jia Ji of UB 20

Huang Lian E Jiao Tang

Primary: 20, 95, 465, 660, 727, 728, 776, 787, 800, 802, 880, 1550, 1800, 2489, 2720, 10000

Secondary: 7.83, 120, 166, 428, 430, 440, 444, 464, 470, 600, 620, 624, 625, 650, 690, 784, 832, 840, 1489, 1500, 1600, 1850, 1865, 2008, 2128, 2213, 2950, 3000, 5000, 6000

Tertiary: 1.1, 1.2, 3.5, 7.69, 9.19, 10, 28, 35, 46.5, 60, 72, 73, 100, 125, 141, 200, 224, 275, 304, 342, 467, 476, 524, 528, 574, 629, 664, 666, 712, 734, 745, 747, 766, 786, 854, 866, 875, 885, 962, 1000, 1614, 2127, 2170, 5148

Suggested points:
DU 14
Jia Ji of UB 23

Huang Lian Jie Du Tang

Primary: 20, 95, 660, 727, 776, 787, 802, 880, 1550, 10000

Secondary: 9.19, 146, 160, 320, 440, 464, 465, 522, 728, 766, 832, 952, 1489, 1500, 1800, 2489, 2720, 2950, 5000

Tertiary: 46.5, 72, 125, 141, 200, 342, 428, 444, 467, 476, 574, 629, 664, 666, 682, 690, 712, 734, 741, 745, 747, 784, 875, 885, 962, 987, 1000, 1234, 1600, 1614, 1862, 1865, 2050, 2128, 2688

Suggested points:
DU 14
Jia Ji of UB 20

Huo Xiang Zheng Qi Tang

Primary: 20, 72, 95, 120, 125, 146, 440, 444, 464, 465, 522, 666 , 727, 776, 787, 802, 880, 1550, 5000, 10000

Secondary: 160, 304, 320, 600, 660, 683, 688, 690, 728, 766, 800, 832, 952, 1234, 2008, 2489, 2720, 3000, 7344

Tertiary: 1.2, 3, 4.9, 40, 80, 190, 250, 650, 664, 741, 987, 1552, 1600, 1800, 1862, 1865, 2050, 2127, 2128, 2688, 6000

Suggested points:
DU 14
Jia Ji of UB 20

Jiao Ai Tang

Primary: 20, 40, 95, 120, 125, 464, 465, 666, 727, 728, 776, 787, 800, 802, 880, 1550, 2720, 5000, 10000

Secondary: 72, 250, 440, 600, 690, 760, 784, 786, 1600, 2008, 2489, 3000

Tertiary: 1.2, 9.39, 28, 80, 304, 428, 444, 488, 660, 676, 1865, 2127, 2128, 3176, 6000

Suggested points:
Jia Ji of UB 17
Jia Ji of UB 18

Ji Chuan Jian

Primary: 20, 72, 95, 120, 125, 440, 444, 465, 600, 625, 650, 660, 666, 690, 727, 728, 776, 787, 800, 802, 880, 1550, 1600, 2008, 2127, 2489, 2720, 3000, 5000, 10000

Secondary: 1.2, 9.39, 10, 28, 40, 80, 100, 166, 250, 304, 430, 464, 470, 620, 624, 840, 1500, 1800, 1850, 1865, 2050, 2112, 2128, 2213, 5500

Tertiary: 7.69, 9.6, 35, 60, 73, 146, 160, 224, 240, 275, 522, 524, 760, 784, 786, 854, 866, 1234, 2170, 2250, 5148, 6000

Suggested points:
Jia Ji of UB 18
Du 4

Jin Gui Shen Qi Wan

Primary: 20, 72, 95, 120, 125, 146, 440, 444, 464, 465, 522, 600, 625, 650, 660, 666, 690, 727, 728, 776, 787, 800, 802, 880, 1500, 1550, 2008, 2050, 2127, 2128, 2720, 5000, 10000

Secondary: 10, 100, 160, 166, 320, 430, 470, 620, 624, 840, 952, 1234, 1600, 1850, 1865, 2112, 2213, 2250, 2489, 3000, 5500

Tertiary: 1.2, 7.69, 9.39, 28, 35, 40, 60, 73, 224, 275, 524, 682, 741, 784, 786, 854, 866, 987, 1800, 1862, 2170, 2688, 5148, 7344

Suggested points:
Jia Ji of UB 20
Jia Ji of UB 23

Jin Suo Gu Jing Wan

Primary: 20, 40, 72, 95, 120, 125, 440, 444, 465, 600, 625, 650, 660, 666, 690, 727, 728, 776, 787, 800, 802, 880, 1500, 1550, 2008, 2127, 2720, 10000

Secondary: 10, 28, 60, 100, 146, 166, 430, 470, 620, 624, 784, 840, 1600, 1850, 1865, 2050, 2112, 2128, 2213, 2489, 3000, 5000, 5500

Tertiary: 1.2, 7.69, 8, 9.39, 35, 73, 224, 250, 275, 464, 522, 524, 751, 786, 854, 866, 1234, 1800, 2170, 2250, 5148

Suggested points:
Jia Ji of UB 23
DU 4

Juan Bi Tang

Primary: 20, 72, 125, 304, 440, 727, 728, 766, 776, 787, 802, 880, 1550, 2489, 5000, 10000

Secondary: 1.2, 7.83, 10, 40, 80, 95, 120, 146, 160, 240, 250, 428, 444, 450, 464, 465, 600, 625, 650, 660, 666, 676, 683, 688, 690, 800, 1234, 1500, 1600, 1800, 1865, 2008, 2720, 3176, 7344

Tertiary: 1, 8, 9.39, 60, 73, 100, 220, 400, 422, 500, 522, 622, 664, 712, 727.5, 740, 760, 784, 786, 832, 1488, 1552, 1560, 1570, 1850, 1862, 2000, 2112, 2127, 2128, 2250, 3000, 6000

Suggested points:
DU 14
Jia Ji of UB 24

Ju Pi Zhu Ru Tang

Primary: 20, 72, 95, 120, 125, 422, 428, 440, 444, 450, 465, 660, 664, 676, 690, 727, 728, 776, 784, 787, 802, 832, 880, 1500, 1550, 1552, 1600, 1800, 1865, 2008, 2127, 2489, 2720, 5000, 10000

Secondary: 3.9, 4.9, 10, 40, 80, 190, 304, 464, 476, 600, 625, 650, 666, 712, 766, 786, 800, 1000, 1488, 1489, 1850, 2950

Tertiary: 1.2, 2, 7.83, 8, 9.39, 46.5, 60, 73, 100, 141, 160, 200, 220, 240, 250, 342, 400, 424, 432, 500, 574, 622, 629, 648, 688, 700, 727.5, 732, 734, 740, 745, 747, 760, 875, 885, 962, 1234, 1560, 1570, 1614, 1862, 2000, 2112, 2128, 2250, 3000, 3176, 7344

Suggested points:
DU 14
Jia Ji of UB 20

Ling Gui Zhu Gan Tang

Primary: 20, 72, 95, 120, 125, 440, 444, 464, 465, 660, 666, 690, 727, 776, 787, 802, 832, 880, 1550, 1552, 2128, 5000, 10000

Secondary: 10, 146, 160, 190, 304, 320, 422, 522, 664, 728, 766, 784, 800, 952, 1234, 1862, 1865, 2008, 2050, 2127, 2182, 2184, 2189, 2217, 2720, 3672

Tertiary: 4.9, 60, 428, 450, 478, 524, 543, 600, 641, 650, 676, 682, 741, 760, 778, 822, 854, 857, 987, 1050, 1384, 1488, 1744, 2000, 2005, 2030, 2048, 2084, 2100, 2104, 2112, 2116, 2120, 2145, 2160, 2170, 2180, 2489, 2688, 2876, 2950, 3040, 3176, 3524, 3713, 10025, 11780, 17034, 21275

Suggested points:
Jia Ji of UB 20
ST 40

Ling Jiao Gou Teng Tang

Primary: 1.2, 7.83, 10, 20, 72, 125, 727, 787, 802, 880, 10000

Secondary: 9.6, 26, 60, 95, 465, 470, 600, 650, 800, 1550, 1865, 6000

Tertiary: 1.1, 3.5, 4, 4.9, 5.8, 6, 6.3, 7.69, 9.19, 9.39, 28, 35, 73, 100, 120, 166, 224, 275, 430, 440, 444, 464, 522, 524, 624, 625, 660, 666,620, 690, 728, 776, 784, 786, 813, 840, 854, 866, 1500, 1600, 1800, 1850, 2008, 2127, 2128, 2170, 2213, 2489, 2720, 3000, 5000, 5148

Suggested points:
Jia Ji of UB 18
Jia Ji of UB 23

Liu Wei Di Huang Wan

Primary: 20, 465, 660, 727, 728, 776, 787, 802, 880, 1550, 1800, 2489, 2720, 10000

Secondary: 95, 120, 166, 428, 430, 440, 444, 464, 470, 600, 620, 624, 625, 650, 690, 784, 800, 832, 840, 1489, 1500, 1600, 1850, 1865, 2008, 2128, 2213, 2950, 3000, 5000

Tertiary: 1.2, 7.69, 10, 28, 35, 46.5, 60, 72, 100, 125, 141, 200, 224, 275, 304, 342, 467, 476, 524, 528, 574, 629, 664 666, 712, 734, 745, 747, 766, 786, 854, 866, 875, 885, 962, 1000, 1614, 2127, 2170, 5148

Suggested points:
DU 14
Jia Ji of UB 23

Li Zhong Wan

Primary: 20, 72, 95, 125, 440, 465, 727, 787, 802, 880, 1550, 10000

Secondary: 120, 444, 600, 625, 660, 664, 666, 690, 832, 1865, 2008, 2127, 2720, 5000, 5500

Tertiary: 2, 4.9, 9.39, 10, 40, 73, 100, 146, 190, 424, 522, 650, 728, 776, 800, 1234, 1500, 1552, 2050, 2112, 2250

Suggested points:
Jia Ji of UB 20
Du 4

Long Dan Xie Gan Tang

Primary: 20, 660, 727, 776, 787, 802, 880, 1550, 10000

Secondary: 146, 160, 320, 440, 464, 465, 522, 728, 766, 832, 952, 1489, 1500, 1800, 2489 2720, 2950, 5000

Tertiary: 46.5, 72, 95, 125, 141, 200, 342, 428, 444, 467, 476, 574, 629, 664, 666, 682, 690, 712, 734, 741, 745, 747, 784, 875, 885, 962, 987, 1000, 1234, 1600, 1614, 1862, 1865, 2050, 2128, 2688

Suggested points:
DU 14
Jia Ji of UB 20

Ma Huang Tang

Primary: 20, 40, 72, 95, 120, 125, 146, 440, 444, 465, 600, 625, 650, 660, 666, 690, 727, 728, 776, 787, 800, 802, 880, 1234, 1500, 1550, 2008, 2127 2489, 2720, 5000, 7344, 10000

Secondary: 7.83, 9.39, 10, 73, 80, 100, 160, 250, 304, 428, 450, 464, 522, 664, 676, 683, 688, 712, 766, 1600, 1800, 1865, 2112, 2128, 2250, 3000, 3176, 5500

Tertiary: 1.2, 2, 3.9, 8, 60, 220, 240, 400, 422, 424, 500, 622, 727.5, 740, 746, 760, 768, 784, 786, 832, 1000, 1488, 1552, 1560, 1570, 1850, 1862, 2000, 2050

Suggested points:
DU 14
DU 4

Mai Men Dong Tang

Primary: 20, 95, 444, 727, 728, 776, 787, 1550

Secondary: 72, 120, 125, 146, 166, 430, 440, 465, 470, 524, 600, 620, 624, 625, 650, 660, 690, 800, 802, 840, 880, 1234, 1500, 1850, 2008, 2128, 2213, 2720, 3000, 5000, 10000

Tertiary: 0.5, 1.2, 7.69, 7.7, 10, 28, 35, 60, 100, 224, 275, 432, 464, 514, 522, 525, 530, 666, 683, 720, 784, 786, 854, 866, 1600, 1800, 1865, 2127, 2170, 2489, 3702, 5148, 7344

Suggested points:
Jia Ji of UB 13
Jia Ji of UB 23

Ma Xing Shi Gan Tang

Primary: 20, 146, 440, 522, 727, 728, 766, 776, 787, 802, 880, 1234, 1550, 2489, 10000

Secondary: 72, 125, 432, 444, 465, 476, 660, 683, 720, 832, 1489, 1500, 1800, 2720, 2950, 5000, 7344

Tertiary: 0.5, 7.7, 46.5, 95, 141, 200, 304, 342, 428, 514, 524, 525, 530, 574, 629, 650, 664, 688, 712, 734, 745, 747, 784, 800, 875, 885, 962, 1000, 1600, 1614, 1865, 3702

Suggested points:
DU 14
Jia Ji of UB 13

Ma Xing Yi Gan Tang

Primary: 20, 146, 440, 522, 660, 727, 766, 776, 787, 802, 880, 1550, 2489 5000, 10000

Secondary: 72, 125, 160, 320, 444, 464, 465, 683, 688, 728, 832, 952, 1234, 1489, 1500, 1800, 2720, 2950, 7344

Tertiary: 95, 141, 200, 304, 342, 428, 467, 476, 574, 629, 650, 664, 666, 682, 690, 712, 734, 741, 745, 747, 784, 800, 875, 885, 962, 987, 1000, 1600, 1614, 1862, 1865, 2050, 2128, 2688

Suggested points:
DU 14
Jia Ji of SP 20

Ma Zi Ren Wan

Primary: 20, 95, 120, 464, 465, 600, 650, 660, 666, 690, 727, 728, 776, 787, 800, 802, 880, 1550, 1600, 1800, 2008, 2489, 2720, 3000, 5000, 10000

Secondary: 1.2, 28, 125, 166, 304, 428, 430, 440, 444, 470, 620, 624, 625, 784, 832, 840, 1489, 1500, 1850, 1865, 2127, 2128, 2213, 2950

Tertiary: 7.69, 9.6, 10, 35, 40, 46.5, 60, 72, 80, 100, 141, 200, 224, 240, 250, 275, 342, 476, 467, 524, 528, 574, 629, 664, 712, 734, 745, 747, 760, 766, 786, 854, 866, 875, 885, 962, 1000, 1614, 2170, 5148, 6000

Suggested points:
Du 14
Jia Ji of UB 23

Mu Li San

Primary: 10, 20, 72, 95, 120, 125, 440, 444, 464, 465, 600, 625, 650, 660, 666, 690, 727, 728, 776, 787, 800, 802, 880, 1500, 1550, 1600, 1850, 1865, 2008, 2128, 2489, 2720, 3000, 5000, 10000

Secondary: 1.2, 8, 40, 60, 80, 100, 166, 240, 304, 428, 430, 450, 470, 620, 624, 676, 760, 784, 786, 832, 840, 1800, 2000, 2112, 2127

Tertiary: 7.69, 7.83, 9.39, 28, 35, 73, 160, 220, 224, 250, 275, 400, 422, 500, 524, 622, 664, 688, 712, 727.5, 740, 766, 854, 866, 1234, 1488, 1552, 1560, 1570, 1862, 2170, 2213, 2250, 3040, 3176, 5148, 7344

Suggested points:
Jia Ji of UB 13
Jia Ji of UB 23

Nuan Gan Jian

Primary: 20, 95, 125, 600, 666, 690, 727, 776, 787, 802, 880, 1550, 2008, 2720, 10000

Secondary: 9.39, 40, 72, 80, 120, 250, 440, 465, 625, 650, 728, 800, 1600, 2127, 2489, 3000, 5500

Tertiary: 1.2, 73, 100, 146, 160, 304, 444, 464, 522, 660, 1234, 1500, 2050, 2112, 2250, 5000, 6000

Suggested points:
DU 4
Jia Ji of UB 18

Ping Wei San

Primary: 20, 72, 95, 125, 727, 787, 802, 832, 880, 1550, 10000

Secondary: 422, 440, 444, 465, 5000

Tertiary: 4.9, 120, 190, 664, 1552, 1865

Suggested points:
Jia Ji of ST 20
Jia Ji of ST 21

Pu Ji Xiao Du Yin

Primary: 20, 727, 776, 787, 802, 880, 1550, 2489, 10000

Secondary: 440, 465, 476, 522, 660, 728, 766, 832, 1489, 1800, 2720, 2950, 5000

Tertiary: 46.5, 72, 125, 141, 146, 200, 304, 342, 428, 574, 629, 650, 664, 683, 688, 712, 734, 745, 747, 784, 800, 875, 885, 962, 1000, 1234, 1500, 1600, 1614, 1865, 7344

Suggested points:
DU 14
GB 20

Qiang Huo Sheng Shi Tang

Primary: 20, 727, 727, 776, 787, 802, 880, 1550

Secondary: 125, 146, 160, 320, 440, 464, 522, 952, 5000, 6000, 10000

Tertiary: 72, 95, 240, 304, 444, 660, 666, 682, 690, 728, 741, 766, 987, 1234, 1500, 1862, 2050, 2128, 2688

Suggested points:
DU 14
Jia Ji of UB 20

Qi Ju Di Huang Wan

Primary: 20, 95, 120, 166, 430, 444, 465, 470, 600, 620, 624, 625, 650, 660, 690, 727, 728, 776, 787, 800, 802, 840, 880, 1550, 1850, 2008, 2128, 2213, 2720, 3000, 5000, 10000

Secondary: 1.2, 7.69, 10, 28, 35, 60, 72, 100, 125, 224, 275, 440, 464, 524, 666, 784, 786, 854, 866, 1500, 1600, 1800, 1865, 2127, 2170, 2489, 5148

Tertiary: 8, 9.6, 23.2, 33, 80.9, 110, 112, 143, 190, 212, 218, 240, 241.68, 242, 246, 300, 303, 304, 304.6, 305, 317, 428, 484, 528, 680, 742.4, 760, 832, 2000, 2003, 2013, 2050, 2088.59, 2112, 2252.8, 2358, 2466.9, 2467, 3040, 3056.9, 3057, 19180.5, 23570.5

Suggested points:
Jia Ji of UB 18
Jia Ji of UB 23

Qing Gu San

Primary: 20, 465, 660, 727, 728, 776, 787, 802, 880, 1550, 2720, 10000

Secondary: 95, 120, 166, 428, 430, 440, 444, 464, 470, 600, 620, 624, 625, 650, 690, 784, 800, 832, 840, 1500, 1600, 1800, 1850, 1865, 2008, 2128, 2213 2489, 3000, 5000

Tertiary: 1.2, 7.69, 10, 28, 35, 46.5, 60, 72, 100, 125, 141, 200, 224, 275, 304, 342, 467, 476, 524, 528, 574, 629, 664, 666, 712, 734, 745, 747, 766, 786, 854, 866, 875, 885, 962, 1000, 1489, 1614, 2127, 2170, 2950, 5148

Suggested points:
DU 14
Jia Ji of UB 23

Qing Hao Bie Jia Tang

Primary: 20, 465, 660, 727, 728, 776, 787, 802, 880, 1550, 2720, 10000

Secondary: 95, 120, 166, 428, 430, 440, 444, 464, 470, 600, 620, 624, 625, 650, 690, 784, 800, 832, 840, 1500, 1600, 1800, 1850, 1865, 2008, 2128, 2213, 2489, 3000, 5000

Tertiary: 1.2, 7.69, 10, 28, 35, 46.5, 60, 72, 100, 125, 141, 200, 224, 275, 304, 342, 467, 476, 524, 528, 574, 629, 664, 666, 712, 734, 745, 747, 766, 786, 854, 866, 875, 885, 962, 1000, 1489, 1614, 2170, 2950, 5148

Suggested points:
DU 14
Jia Ji of UB 23

Qing Qi Hua Tan Wan

Primary: 20, 95, 125, 465, 660, 727, 728, 766, 776, 785, 787, 802, 832, 880, 1234, 1500, 1550, 2489, 2720, 2950, 10000

Secondary: 72, 146, 304, 428, 432, 440, 444, 450, 464, 522, 524, 650, 664, 666, 690, 778, 800, 822, 1000, 1488, 1489, 1552, 1600, 1800, 1865, 2008, 2127, 2128, 2182, 2184, 2189, 2217, 3672, 5000

Tertiary: 0.5, 7.7, 10, 46.5, 60, 120, 141, 200, 222, 262, 342, 422, 467, 476, 478, 514, 525, 530, 543, 552, 574, 656, 665, 676, 683, 712, 720, 731, 732, 734, 745, 747, 760, 854, 857, 875, 885, 962, 1050, 1384, 1614, 1744, 2000, 2005, 2030, 2048, 2050, 2084, 2100, 2104, 2112, 2116, 2120, 2145, 2160, 2170, 2180, 2876, 3040, 3176, 3524, 3702, 3713, 7344, 10025, 11780, 17034, 21275

Suggested points:
Jia Ji of UB 13
Jia Ji of UB 20

Qing Wei San

Primary: 20, 95, 465, 660, 727, 728, 776, 787, 802, 880, 1550, 1800, 2489, 2720, 10000

Secondary: 9.19, 120, 166, 428, 430, 440, 444, 464, 470, 600, 620, 624, 625, 650, 690, 784, 800, 832, 840, 1489, 1500, 1600, 1850, 1865, 2008, 2128, 2213, 2950, 3000, 5000

Tertiary: 1.2, 7.69, 10, 28, 35, 46.5, 60, 72, 100, 125, 141, 200, 224, 275, 304, 342, 467, 476, 524, 528, 574, 629, 664, 666, 712, 734, 745, 747, 766, 786, 854, 866, 875, 885, 962, 1000, 1614, 2127, 2170, 5148

Suggested points:
DU 14
Jia Ji of UB 23

Qing Ying Tang

Primary: 20, 95, 120, 464, 600, 650, 660, 465, 666, 690, 727, 728, 776, 787, 800, 802, 880, 1550, 1600, 1800, 2008, 2489, 2720, 3000, 5000, 10000

Secondary: 1.2, 28, 125, 166, 304, 428, 430, 440, 444, 470, 620, 624, 625, 784, 832, 840, 1489, 1500, 1850, 1865, 2127, 2128, 2213, 2950

Tertiary: 7.69, 9.6, 10, 35, 40, 46.5, 60, 72, 80, 100, 141, 200, 224, 240, 250, 275, 342, 467, 476, 524, 528, 629, 664, 712, 734, 745, 747, 760, 766, 786, 854, 866, 875, 885, 962, 1000, 1614, 2170, 5148, 6000

Suggested points:
DU 14
Jia Ji of UB 18

Qing Zao Jiu Fei Tang

Primary: 20, 95, 444, 727, 728, 776, 787, 1550

Secondary: 72, 120, 125, 146, 166, 430, 440, 465, 470, 524, 600, 620, 624, 625, 650, 660, 690, 800, 802, 840, 880, 1234, 1500, 1850, 2008, 2128, 2213, 2720, 3000, 5000, 10000

Tertiary: 0.5, 1.2, 7.69, 7.7, 10, 28, 35, 60, 100, 224, 275, 432, 464, 514, 522, 525, 530, 666, 683, 720, 766, 784, 786, 854, 866, 1600, 1800, 1865, 2127, 2170, 2489, 3702, 5148, 7344

Suggested points:
Jia Ji of UB 13
Jia Ji of UB 23

Ren Shen Bai Du San

Primary: 20, 72, 125, 304, 440, 727, 728, 766, 776, 787, 802, 880, 1550, 2489, 5000, 10000

Secondary: 1.2, 7.83, 10, 40, 80, 95, 120, 146, 160, 240, 250, 428, 444, 450, 464, 465, 600, 625, 650, 660, 666, 676, 683, 688, 690, 800, 1234, 1500, 1600, 1800, 1865, 2008, 2720, 3176, 7344

Tertiary: 1, 8, 9.39, 60, 73, 100, 220, 400, 422, 500, 522, 622, 664, 712, 727.5, 740, 760, 784, 786, 832, 1488, 1552, 1560, 1570, 1850, 1862, 2000, 2112, 2127, 2128, 2250, 3000, 6000

Suggested points:
Du 14
Jia Ji of UB 20

Sang Ju Yin

Primary: 20, 146, 440, 465, 522, 727, 728, 766, 776, 787, 802, 880, 1234, 1550, 2489, 10000

Secondary: 72, 125, 432, 444, 660, 683, 720, 832, 1489, 1500, 1800, 2720, 2950, 5000, 7344

Tertiary: 7.7, 46.5, 95, 141, 200, 304, 342, 428, 467, 476, 514, 524, 525, 530, 574, 629, 650, 664, 688, 712, 734, 745, 747, 784, 800, 875, 885, 962, 1000, 1600, 1614, 1865, 3702

Suggested points:
DU 14
Jia Ji of UB 13

Sang Piao Xiao San

Primary: 1.2, 10, 20, 40, 72, 80, 95, 120, 125, 304, 428, 440, 444, 464, 465, 600, 625, 650, 660, 666, 676, 690, 727, 728, 760, 776, 784, 786, 787, 800, 802, 880, 1550, 1600, 1800, 1850, 1865, 2008, 2127, 2128, 2489, 2720, 3000, 5000, 10000

Secondary: 8, 9.39, 28, 60, 100, 160, 166, 240, 250, 430, 450, 470, 500, 620, 624, 664, 688, 740, 832, 840, 1488, 1862, 2000, 2112, 2213, 3176

Tertiary: 7.69, 7.83, 9.6, 35, 47, 73, 220, 224, 275, 400, 422, 424, 524, 622, 712, 727.5, 766, 854, 866, 1234, 1552, 1560, 1570, 2145, 2170, 2250, 3040, 5148, 6000, 7344

Suggested points:
Jia Ji of UB 18
Jia Ji of UB 23

Sang Xing Tang

Primary: 20, 95, 440, 444, 660, 727, 728, 776, 787, 802, 880, 1500, 1550, 1800, 2489, 2720, 10000

Secondary: 72, 120, 125, 146, 166, 428, 430, 432, 522, 524, 600, 620, 624, 625, 650, 690, 766, 784, 800, 832, 840, 1234, 1489, 1600, 1850, 1865, 2008, 2128, 2213, 2950, 3000, 5000

Tertiary: 0.5, 1.2, 7.69, 7.7, 10, 28, 35, 46.5, 60, 100, 141, 200, 224, 275, 304, 342, 514, 525, 528, 530, 574, 629, 664, 666, 683, 712, 720, 734, 745, 747, 786, 854, 866, 875, 885, 962, 1000, 1614, 2127, 2170, 3702, 5148, 7344

Suggested points:
DU 14
Jia Ji of UB 13

San Zi Yang Qin Tang

Primary: 20, 95, 125, 304, 465, 666, 690, 727, 728, 776, 787, 800, 802, 880, 1234, 1550, 2720, 10000

Secondary: 72, 80, 120, 146, 440, 444, 524, 600, 650, 760, 766, 784, 1552, 1600, 2008, 2127, 2128, 2182, 2184, 2189, 2217, 2489, 3000, 3672, 5000

Tertiary: 0.5, 1.2, 7.7, 10, 40, 60, 250, 422, 428, 432, 450, 478, 500, 514, 522, 525, 530, 543, 641, 660, 664, 676, 683, 720, 778, 822, 832, 854, 857, 1050, 1384, 1488, 1500, 1744, 1865, 2000, 2005, 2030, 2048, 2050, 2084, 2100, 2104, 2112, 2116, 2120, 2145, 2160, 2170, 2180, 2876, 2950, 3040, 3176, 3524, 3702, 3713, 6000, 7344, 10025, 11780, 17034, 21275

Suggested points:
DU 14
Jia Ji of UB 13

Shao Fu Zhu Yu Tang

Primary: 20, 95, 666, 727, 776, 787, 802, 880, 1550, 2720, 3000, 10000

Secondary: 1.2, 40, 80, 120, 125, 250, 304, 464, 600, 690, 728, 800, 1600, 2008, 2489, 5000, 6000

Tertiary: 3, 9.39, 9.6, 28, 160, 240, 320, 324, 465, 500, 650, 760, 1800, 2127

Suggested points:
LIV 3
SP 10

Shao Yao Tang

Primary: 20, 727, 776, 787, 802, 880, 1550, 2489, 2720, 10000

Secondary: 95, 304, 464, 465, 476, 660, 666, 728, 800, 832, 1489, 1800, 2950, 3000, 5000

Tertiary: 1.2, 9.39, 40, 46.5, 80, 120, 125, 141, 200, 250, 342, 428, 574, 600, 629, 650, 664, 690, 712, 734, 745, 747, 766, 784, 875, 885, 962, 1000, 1500, 1614, 1865, 2008, 6000

Suggested points:
DU 14
Jia Ji of UB 18

Sheng Hua Tang

Primary: 20, 72, 95, 120, 125, 440, 444, 465, 600, 625, 650, 660, 666, 690, 727, 728, 776, 787, 800, 802, 880, 1550, 1600, 2008, 2127, 2489, 2720, 3000, 5000, 10000

Secondary: 1.2, 9.39, 10, 28, 40, 80, 100, 166, 250, 304, 430, 464, 470, 620, 624, 840, 1500, 1800, 1850, 1865, 2050, 2112, 2128, 2213, 5500

Tertiary: 7.69, 9.6, 35, 60, 73, 146, 160, 224, 240, 275, 522, 524, 760, 784, 786, 854, 866, 1234, 2170, 2250, 5148, 6000

Suggested points:
Jia Ji of UB 18
Jia Ji of UB 23

Sheng Mai San

Primary: 10, 20, 72, 95, 120, 125, 440, 444, 464, 465, 600, 625, 650, 660, 666, 690, 727, 728, 776, 787, 800, 802, 880, 1500, 1550, 1600, 1850, 1865, 2008, 2128, 2489, 2720, 3000, 5000, 10000

Secondary: 1.2, 8, 40, 60, 80, 100, 166, 240, 304, 428, 430, 450, 470, 620,624, 676, 760, 784, 786, 832, 840, 1800, 2000, 2112, 2127, 2213

Tertiary: 7.69, 7.83, 9.39, 28, 35, 73, 160, 220, 224, 250, 275, 400, 422, 500, 524, 622, 664, 688, 712, 727.5, 740, 766, 854, 866, 1234, 1488, 1552, 1560, 1570, 1862, 2170, 2250, 3040, 3176, 5148, 7344

Suggested points:
Jia Ji of UB 15
Jia Ji of UB 23

Shen Ling Bai Zhu San

Primary: 20, 72, 95, 125, 440, 727, 787, 802, 880, 1550, 5000, 10000

Secondary: 120, 146, 160, 320, 444, 464, 465, 522, 660, 776, 832, 952

Tertiary: 4.9, 190, 664, 666, 682, 690, 741, 987, 1234, 1552, 1862, 1865, 2050, 2128, 2688

Suggested points:
Jia Ji of UB 20
Du 4

Shen Tong Zhu Yu Tang

Primary: 20, 727,776, 787, 802, 880, 1550, 10000

Secondary: 1.2, 40, 80, 95, 125, 240, 250, 304, 666, 728, 2720, 3000, 6000

Tertiary: 120, 160, 320, 464, 600, 690, 800, 1600, 1800, 2008, 2489, 5000

Suggested points:
Jia Ji of UB 17
Jia Ji of UB 18

Shi Quan Da Bu Tang

Primary: 10, 20, 72, 95, 100, 120, 125, 440, 444, 464, 465, 600, 625, 650, 660, 664, 666, 690, 727, 728, 776, 786, 787, 800, 802, 832, 880, 1500, 1552, 1600, 1850, 1865, 2112, 2127, 2128, 2489, 2720, 3000, 5000, 10000

Secondary: 1.2, 2, 8, 9.39, 40, 60, 73, 80, 146, 160, 166, 190, 240, 250, 304, 422, 424, 428, 430, 450, 470, 620, 624, 676, 712, 760, 784, 840, 1234, 1800, 2000, 2213, 2250, 5500, 7344

Tertiary: 3.9, 4.9, 7.69, 7.83, 28, 35, 220, 224, 275, 400, 500, 522, 524, 568, 622, 688, 727.5, 740, 766, 854, 866, 1000, 1488, 1560, 1570, 1862, 2170, 3040, 3176, 5148

Suggested points:
Jia Ji of UB 20
Jia Ji of UB 23

Shi Xiao San

Primary: 20, 95, 125, 600, 666, 690, 727, 776, 787, 802, 880, 1550, 2008, 2720, 10000

Secondary: 9.39, 40, 72, 80, 120, 250, 440, 465, 625, 650, 728, 800, 1600, 2127, 2489, 3000, 5500

Tertiary: 1.2, 73, 100, 146, 160, 304, 444, 464, 522, 660, 1234, 1500, 2050, 2112, 2250, 5000, 6000

Suggested points:
Jia Ji of UB 18
Du 4

Si Jun Zi Tang

Primary: 20, 72, 95, 120, 125, 160, 440, 444, 464, 465, 660, 666, 690, 727, 776, 787, 802, 832, 880, 1550, 1865, 5000, 10000

Secondary: 10, 40, 80, 146, 320, 422, 428, 450, 522, 600, 625, 650, 664, 676, 688, 728, 766, 786, 800, 952, 1234, 1500, 1552, 1600, 1862, 2008, 2127, 2128, 2250, 2489, 2720, 7344

Tertiary: 1.2, 2, 4.9, 7.83, 8, 9.39, 60, 73, 100, 190, 220, 240, 250, 304, 400, 424, 500, 622, 682, 683, 712, 727.5, 740, 741, 760, 784, 987, 1488, 1560, 1570, 1800, 1850, 2000, 2050, 2112, 2688, 3000, 3176

Suggested points:
Jia Ji of UB 20
Du 4

Si Ni San

Primary: 20, 72, 125, 440, 465, 727, 787, 802, 880, 1550, 5000, 10000

Secondary: 7.83, 26, 95, 444, 776, 800, 832, 1234, 1552

Tertiary: 1.1, 3.5, 4.9, 73, 120, 146, 190, 522, 600, 660, 664, 683, 688, 766, 1865, 2489, 6000, 7344

Suggested points:
DU 14
Jia Ji of UB 20
or
Jia Ji of UB 18
Jia Ji of UB 20

Si Shen Wan

Primary: 20, 72, 95, 125, 440, 465, 727, 787, 802, 880, 1550, 10000

Secondary: 120, 444, 600, 625, 660, 664, 666, 690, 832, 1865, 2008, 2127, 2720, 5000, 5500

Tertiary: 2, 4.9, 9.39, 10, 40, 73, 100, 146, 190, 424, 522, 650, 728, 776, 800, 1234, 1500, 1552, 2050, 2112, 2250

Suggested points:
Jia Ji of UB 20
DU 4

Si Wu Tang

Primary: 20, 95, 120, 464, 465, 666, 727, 728, 776, 787, 800, 802, 880, 1550, 2720, 5000, 10000

Secondary: 26, 40, 125, 600, 690, 760, 786, 2008, 2489, 3000, 6000

Tertiary: 1.1, 1.2, 3.5, 7.83, 9.39, 73, 80, 250, 304, 428, 660, 676, 784, 1600, 2127, 2128, 3176

Suggested points:
Jia Ji of UB 17
Jia Ji of UB 18

Suan Zao Ren Tang

Primary: 20, 95, 120, 428, 464, 465, 660, 690, 727, 728, 776, 784, 786, 787, 800, 802, 880, 1550, 1800, 1865, 2008, 2128, 2489, 2720, 5000, 10000

Secondary: 7.83, 72, 125, 166, 430, 440, 444, 470, 600, 620, 624, 625, 650, 664, 666, 760, 832, 840, 1488, 1489, 1500, 1600, 1850, 2127, 2213, 2950, 3000, 6000

Tertiary: 1.1, 1.2, 3.5, 7.69, 10, 28, 35, 40, 46.5, 60, 73, 100, 141, 200, 224, 275, 304, 342, 450, 467, 476, 524, 528, 574, 629, 676, 712, 734, 745, 747, 766, 854, 866, 875, 885, 962, 1000, 1614, 2000, 2112, 2170, 3176, 5148

Suggested points:
DU 14
Jia Ji of UB 17

Su Zi Jiang Qi Tang

Primary: 20, 72, 95, 120, 125, 146, 440, 444, 465, 666, 690, 727, 728, 776, 787, 800, 802, 822, 880, 1234, 1550, 2008, 2127, 2720, 3672, 10000

Secondary: 4.7, 10, 100, 128, 172, 263, 304, 322, 411, 434, 487, 515, 521, 522, 524, 600, 625, 633, 650, 660, 664, 665, 712, 756, 766, 782, 784, 871, 886, 890, 1233, 1283, 1500, 1552, 1865, 2050, 2112, 2128, 2182, 2184, 2189, 2217, 2489, 3124, 3125, 5500, 7344, 7346

Tertiary: 0.5, 7.7, 9.39, 40, 60, 73, 80, 422, 428, 432, 450, 464, 478, 514, 525, 530, 543, 641, 676, 683, 760, 778, 832, 854, 857, 1000, 1050, 1384, 1488, 1600, 1744, 2000, 2005, 2030, 2048, 2084, 2100, 2104, 2116, 2120, 2145, 2160, 2170, 2180, 2250, 2876, 2950, 3000, 3040, 3176, 3524, 3702, 3713, 5000, 9999, 10025, 11780, 17034, 21275

Suggested points:
Jia Ji of UB 13
DU 4

Tian Ma Gou Teng Yin

Primary: 1.2, 7.83, 10, 20, 72, 95, 120, 125, 465, 470, 600, 650, 660, 666, 690, 727, 728, 776, 784, 787, 800, 802, 880, 1500, 1550, 1600, 1800, 1865, 2008, 2489, 2720, 3000, 5000, 6000, 10000

Secondary: 1.1, 3.5, 9.39, 9.6, 26, 28, 46.5, 60, 73, 141, 166, 200, 304, 342, 428, 430, 440, 444, 467, 476, 522, 574, 620, 624, 625, 629, 664, 712, 734, 745, 747, 766, 832, 840, 875, 885, 962, 1000, 1489, 1614, 1850, 2127, 2128, 2213, 2950

Tertiary: 4, 4.9, 5.8, 6, 6.3, 7.69, 9.19, 35, 40, 80, 100, 224, 240, 250, 275, 524, 528, 760, 786, 813, 854, 866, 2170, 5148

Suggested points:
DU 14
Jia Ji of UB 18

Tian Tai Wu Yao San

Primary: 20, 95, 125, 465, 600, 666, 690, 727, 776, 787, 800, 802, 880, 1550, 2008, 2720, 10000

Secondary: 9.39, 26, 40, 72, 73, 80, 120, 250, 440, 625, 650, 728, 1600, 2127, 2489, 3000, 5500, 6000

Tertiary: 1.1, 1.2, 3.5, 7.83, 100, 146, 160, 304, 444, 464, 522, 660, 1234, 1500, 2050, 2112, 2250, 5000

Suggested points:
Jia Ji of UB 18
DU 4

Tian Wang Bu Xin Dan

Primary: 20, 95, 120, 125, 428, 440, 464, 465, 660, 727, 728, 776, 784, 786, 787, 800, 802, 880, 1500, 1550, 1600, 1800, 1865, 2008, 2128, 2489, 2720, 5000, 6000, 10000

Secondary: 7.83, 10, 40, 72, 304, 600, 664, 666, 690, 760, 832, 840, 1488, 1489, 1850, 2112, 2127, 2213, 2950, 3000

Tertiary: 1.1, 1.2, 3.5, 3.9, 7.69, 28, 35, 46.5, 60, 73, 100, 141, 200, 212, 224, 240, 275, 342, 424, 444, 450, 467, 476, 524, 528, 574, 625, 629, 650, 676, 712, 734 ,745, 747, 766, 854, 866, 875, 885, 962, 1000, 1614, 2000, 2170, 3176, 5148

Suggested points:
Jia Ji of UB 15 (or Du 14 if heat is excessive)
Jia Ji of UB 17

Tiao Wei Cheng Qi Tang

Primary: 20, 727, 776, 787, 802, 880, 1550, 2489, 2720, 10000

Secondary: 95, 304, 464, 465, 660, 666, 728, 800, 832, 1489, 1600, 1800, 2950, 3000, 5000

Tertiary: 1.2, 40, 46.5, 80, 120, 125, 141, 200, 250, 342, 428, 467, 476, 574, 600, 629, 650, 664, 690, 712, 734, 745, 747, 766, 784, 875, 885, 962, 1000, 1500, 1614, 1865, 2008, 6000

Suggested points:
DU 14
Jia Ji of UB 18

Tong Xie Yao Fang

Primary: 20, 72, 95, 125, 440, 465, 727, 787, 832, 880, 1550, 5000, 10000

Secondary: 26, 120, 146, 160, 320, 444, 464, 522, 660, 776, 952

Tertiary: 1.1, 3.5, 4.9, 7.83, 73, 190, 664, 666, 682, 690, 741, 800, 832, 987, 1234, 1552, 1862, 1865, 2050, 2128, 2688, 6000

Suggested points:
Jia Ji of UB 18
Jia Ji of UB 20

Wan Dai Tang

Primary: 20, 72, 95, 125, 440, 727, 787, 802, 880, 1550, 5000, 10000

Secondary: 120, 146, 160, 320, 444, 464, 465, 522, 660, 776, 832, 952

Tertiary: 4.9, 190, 664, 666, 682, 690, 741, 987, 1234, 1552, 1862, 1865, 2050, 2128, 2688

Suggested points:
Jia Ji of UB 20
Du 4

Wen Dan Tang

Primary: 20, 72, 95, 120, 125, 304, 465, 666, 690, 727, 728,, 776, 787, 800, 802, 832, 880, 1550, 1552, 1865, 2008, 2127, 2720, 5000, 10000

Secondary: 10, 80, 190, 422, 440, 444, 464, 600, 650, 660, 664, 760, 784, 1600, 2128, 2182, 2184, 2189, 2217 2489, 3000, 3524

Tertiary: 1.2, 3, 4.9, 40, 60, 250, 428, 450, 478, 500, 524, 543, 641, 676, 766, 778, 822, 854, 857, 1050, 1234, 1384, 1488, 1744, 2000, 2005, 2030, 2048, 2050, 2084, 2100, 2104, 2112, 2116, 2120, 2145, 2160, 2170, 2180, 2876, 2950, 3040, 3176, 3672, 3713, 6000, 10025, 11780, 17034

Suggested points:
Jia Ji of UB 18
Jia Ji of UB 20

Wen Jing Tang

Primary: 20, 40, 95, 120, 125, 465, 600, 666, 690, 727, 728, 776, 787, 800, 802, 880, 1550, 2008, 2127, 2489, 2720, 10000

Secondary: 9.39, 72, 80, 250, 440, 444, 464, 625, 650, 660, 760, 786, 1600, 2112, 2128, 3000, 5000, 5500

Tertiary: 1.2, 73, 100, 146, 160, 304, 424, 428, 522, 664, 676, 784, 1234, 1488, 1500, 1865, 2050, 2250, 3176, 6000

Suggested points:
Jia Ji of UB 17
Du 4

Wu Ling San

Primary: 20, 72, 95, 120, 125, 146, 160, 440, 444, 464, 465, 522, 600, 660, 666, 690, 727, 728, 776, 787, 802, 880, 1550, 2008, 2127, 2720, 5000, 10000

Secondary: 9.39, 40, 80, 250, 320, 625, 650, 664, 800, 832, 952, 1234, 1500, 1600, 1865, 2050, 2128, 2250, 2489, 3000, 5500

Tertiary: 1.2, 2, 3, 4.9, 10, 73, 100, 190, 304, 424, 682, 741, 1552, 1862, 2112, 2688, 6000, 7344

Suggested points:
Jia Ji of UB 20
Du 4

Wu Pi San

Primary: 20, 72, 95, 120, 125, 440, 464, 666, 727, 776, 787, 802, 880, 1550, 5000, 10000

Secondary: 146, 160, 320, 444, 465, 522, 600, 660, 690, 728, 832, 952, 2008, 2720, 3000

Tertiary: 1.2, 3, 4.9, 40, 80, 190, 250, 304, 664, 682, 741, 800, 987, 1234, 1552, 1600, 1862, 1865, 2050, 2127, 2128, 2489, 2688, 6000

Suggested points:
Jia Ji of UB 18
Jia Ji of UB 20

Wu Wei Xiao Du Yin

Primary: 20, 95, 465, 727, 776, 787, 802, 880, 1550, 1600, 1800, 2720, 10000

Secondary: 9.19, 432, 625, 660, 664, 673, 676, 728, 758, 832, 884, 885, 1000, 1455, 1489, 1500, 2016, 2489, 2950

Tertiary: 3, 46.5, 141, 146, 200, 254, 342, 345, 428, 440, 444, 467, 476, 495, 522, 574, 610, 615, 629, 690, 712, 734, 745, 747, 766, 784, 785, 790, 797, 800, 846, 864, 875, 920, 962, 1520, 1614, 1865, 2050, 2170, 7989

Suggested points:
Du 14
Jia Ji of UB 17

Wu Zhu Yu Tang

Primary: 20, 72, 95, 125, 440, 465, 664, 690, 727, 787, 802, 832, 880, 1550, 2008, 2127, 10000

Secondary: 3.9, 4.9, 120, 190, 422, 444, 600, 625, 660, 666, 1552, 1865, 2720, 5000, 5500

Tertiary: 2, 9.39, 10, 40, 73, 100, 146, 424, 450, 522, 650, 676, 728, 776, 784, 800, 1234, 1500, 2050, 2112, 2250

Suggested points:
Jia Ji of UB 20
Du 4

Xiao Chai Hu Tang

Primary: 20, 72, 120, 125, 440, 444, 465, 727, 776, 787, 802, 832, 880, 1550, 5000, 10000

Secondary: 95, 146, 428, 522, 600, 660, 676, 688, 728, 760, 766, 786, 800, 1552, 1800, 1865, 2489, 2720, 3176

Tertiary: 4.9, 190, 304, 333, 422, 450, 664, 666, 683, 690, 1234, 1488, 1500, 1600, 2008, 2128, 7344

Suggested points:
Jia Ji of UB 13
Jia Ji of UB 20

Xiao Cheng Qi Tang

Primary: 20, 727, 776, 787, 802, 880, 1550, 2489, 2720, 10000

Secondary: 95, 304, 464, 465, 660, 666, 728, 800, 832, 1489, 1600, 1800, 2950, 3000, 5000

Tertiary: 1.2, 40, 46.5, 80, 120, 125, 141, 200, 250, 342, 428, 467, 476, 574, 600, 629, 650, 664, 690, 712, 734, 745, 747, 766, 784, 875, 885, 962, 1000, 1500, 1614, 1865, 2008, 6000

Suggested points:
DU 14
Jia Ji of UB 18

Xiao Feng San

Primary: 20, 146, 440, 522, 660, 727, 766, 776, 787, 802, 880, 1550, 2489, 5000, 10000

Secondary: 72, 125, 160, 320, 444, 464, 465, 683, 688, 728, 832, 952, 1234, 1489, 1500, 1800, 2720, 2950, 7344

Tertiary: 46.5, 95, 141, 200, 304, 342, 428, 467, 476, 574, 629, 650, 664, 666, 682, 690, 712, 734, 741, 745, 747, 784, 800, 875, 885, 962, 987, 1000, 1600, 1614, 1862, 1865, 2050, 2128

Suggested points:
DU 14
Jia Ji of UB 20

Xiao Jian Zhong Tang

Primary: 20, 40, 72, 95, 120, 125, 428, 440, 444, 464, 465, 600, 660, 664, 666, 676, 690, 727, 728, 776, 786, 787, 800, 802, 832, 880, 1550, 1865, 2008 2720, 5000, 10000

Secondary: 9.39, 10, 80, 422, 424, 450, 625, 650, 688, 740, 760, 784, 1488, 1500, 1552, 1600, 1862, 2000, 2112, 2127, 2128, 2489

Tertiary: 1.2, 2, 4.9, 7.83, 8, 47, 60, 73, 100, 160, 190, 220, 240, 250, 304, 400, 500, 622, 712, 727.5, 766, 1234, 1560, 1570, 1800, 1850, 2145, 2250, 3000, 3176, 7344

Suggested points:
Jia Ji of UB 17
Jia Ji of UB 20

Xiao Qing Long Tang

Primary: 20, 72, 95, 120, 125, 146, 440, 444, 465, 600, 660, 683, 727, 728, 766, 776, 787, 802, 832, 880, 1234, 1500, 1550, 1865, 2489, 5000, 7344, 10000

Secondary: 7.83, 10, 40, 80, 304, 422, 428, 432, 450, 464, 522, 625, 650, 664, 666, 676, 688, 690, 720, 800, 1552, 1600, 1800, 2008, 2127, 2720, 3176

Tertiary: 0.5, 1.2, 2, 4.9, 7.7, 8, 9.39, 60, 73, 100, 160, 190, 220, 240, 250, 400, 424, 500, 514, 524, 525, 530, 622, 712, 727.5, 740, 760, 784, 786, 1488, 1560, 1570, 1850, 1862, 2000, 2112, 2128, 2250, 3000, 3702

Suggested points:
Jia Ji of UB 13
Jia Ji of UB 20

Xiao Yao San

Primary: 20, 95, 120, 125, 465, 727, 786, 787, 800, 802, 880, 1550, 5000, 10000

Secondary: 26, 72, 440, 444, 464, 660, 664, 728, 832, 1865, 2720

Tertiary: 1.1, 3.5, 4.9, 7.83, 40, 73, 190, 424, 428, 600, 666, 676, 690, 760, 776, 784, 1488, 1552, 2008, 2127, 2128, 2489, 3176, 6000

Suggested points:
Jia Ji of UB 18
Jia Ji of UB 20

Xie Bai San

Primary: 20, 727, 766, 787, 1550

Secondary: 146, 432, 440, 465, 522, 660, 728, 766, 802, 832, 880, 1234, 1489, 1500, 1800, 2489, 2720, 2950, 10000

Tertiary: 0.5, 7.7, 46.5, 72, 95, 125, 141, 200, 342, 428, 444, 467, 476, 514, 524, 525, 530, 574, 629, 664, 683, 712, 720, 734, 745, 747, 784, 875, 885, 962, 1000, 1600, 1614, 1865, 3702, 7344

Suggested points:
DU 14
Jia Ji of UB 13

Xie Xin Tang

Primary: 20, 95, 464, 660, 666, 727, 728, 776, 787, 802, 880, 1550, 2489 2720, 5000, 10000

Secondary: 120, 125, 146, 160, 304, 320, 440, 465, 522, 690, 766, 800, 832, 952, 1489, 1500, 1600, 1800, 2008, 2950, 3000

Tertiary: 1.2, 40, 46.5, 72, 80, 141, 250, 342, 428, 444, 467, 476, 574, 600, 629, 650, 664, 682, 712, 734, 741, 745, 747, 784, 875, 885, 962, 987, 1000, 1234, 1614, 1862, 1865, 2050, 2128, 2688, 6000

Suggested points:
DU 14
Jia Ji of UB 20

Xi Jiao Di Huang Tang

Primary: 20, 95, 120, 125, 444, 465, 600, 625, 666, 690, 727, 728, 776, 787, 800, 802, 880, 1550, 1600, 1800, 2008, 2489, 2720, 3000, 5000, 10000

Secondary: 1.2, 3, 9.19, 28, 72, 166, 304, 430, 440, 464, 470, 620, 624, 650, 660, 673, 676, 758, 840, 884, 1455, 1500, 1850, 2016, 2050 2127, 2128, 2170, 2213

Tertiary: 7.69, 9.6, 10, 35, 40, 60, 80, 100, 146, 224, 240, 250, 254, 275, 345, 432, 484, 495, 500, 524, 610, 615, 760, 784, 786, 790, 797, 832, 854, 864, 866, 885, 920, 1520, 1865, 5148, 6000

Suggested points:
DU 14
Jia Ji of UB 18

Xing Su San

Primary: 20, 72, 95, 125, 440, 444, 524, 727, 728, 776, 787, 1234, 1550

Secondary: 10, 60, 100, 120, 146, 304, 428, 464, 465, 600, 650, 660, 666, 690, 760, 766, 784, 800, 802, 832, 854, 866, 880, 1500, 1600, 1865, 2000, 2008, 2050, 2112, 2127, 2128, 2170, 2489, 2720, 3000, 3040, 5000, 10000

Tertiary: 0.5, 1.2, 7.69, 7.7, 28, 35, 166, 190, 224, 275, 422, 430, 432, 450, 470, 478, 514, 522, 525, 530, 543, 620, 624, 625, 641, 664, 676, 683, 720, 778, 786, 822, 840, 857, 1050, 1384, 1488, 1552, 1744, 1800, 1850, 2005, 2030, 2048, 2084, 2100, 2104, 2116, 2120, 2145, 2160, 2180, 2182, 2184, 2189, 2213, 2217, 2876, 2950, 3176, 3524, 3672, 3702, 3713, 5148, 7344, 10025, 11780, 17034, 21275

Suggested points:
DU 14
Jia ji of UB 13

Xue Fu Zhu Yu Tang

Primary: 727, 787, 880, 10000

Secondary: 20, 26, 95, 666, 776, 800, 802, 1550, 2720, 3000, 6000

Tertiary: 1.2, 40, 80, 120, 125, 250, 304, 464, 465, 600, 690, 728, 1600, 2008, 2489, 5000

Suggested points:
Jia Ji of UB 17
Jia Ji of UB 18

Yi Guan Jian

Primary: 465, 727, 787, 800, 802, 880, 1550, 10000

Secondary: 20, 26, 95, 120, 166, 430, 444, 470, 600, 620, 624, 625, 650, 660, 690, 728, 776, 840, 1850, 2008, 2128, 2213, 2720, 3000, 5000

Tertiary: 1.1, 1.2, 3.5, 7.69, 7.83, 10, 28, 35, 60, 72, 73, 100, 125, 224, 275, 440, 464, 524, 666, 784, 786, 854, 866, 1500, 1600, 1800, 1865, 2127, 2170, 2489, 5148, 6000

Suggested points:
Jia Ji of UB 18
Jia Ji of UB 23

Yin Chen Hao Tang

Primary: 20, 146, 727, 776, 787, 802, 880, 1550, 10000

Secondary: 72, 95, 125, 160, 320, 440, 444, 464, 465, 522, 615, 625, 673, 676, 690, 758, 884, 952, 1455, 1600, 1800, 2016, 2050, 2720, 5000

Tertiary: 3, 254, 345, 495, 597, 610, 660, 666, 682, 728, 741, 790, 797, 864, 885, 920, 987, 1234, 1500, 1520, 1862, 2128, 2170, 2688, 7989

Suggested points:
DU 14
Jia Ji of UB 20

Yin Qiao San

Primary: 20, 727, 776, 787, 802, 880, 1550, 2489, 10000

Secondary: 440, 465, 522, 660, 728, 766, 832, 1489, 1800, 2720, 2950, 5000

Tertiary: 46.5, 72, 125, 141, 146, 200, 304, 342, 428, 467, 476, 574, 629, 650, 664, 683, 688, 712, 734, 745, 747, 784, 800, 875, 885, 962, 1000, 1234, 1500, 1600, 1614, 1865, 7344

Suggested points:
DU 14
Jia Ji of UB 13

You Gui Wan

Primary: 20, 72, 95, 120, 125, 440, 444, 465, 600, 625, 650, 660, 666, 690, 727, 728, 776, 787, 800, 802, 880, 1550, 2008, 2127, 2720, 10000

Secondary: 10, 100, 166, 430, 470, 620, 624, 840, 1500, 1600, 1850, 1865, 2050, 2112, 2128, 2213, 2489, 3000, 5000, 5500

Tertiary: 1.2, 7.69, 9.39, 28, 35, 40, 60, 73, 146, 224, 275, 464, 522, 524, 784, 786, 854, 866, 1234, 1800, 2170, 2250, 5148

Suggested points:
DU 4
Jia Ji of UB 23

You Gui Yin

Primary: 20, 40, 72, 95, 120, 125, 440, 444, 465, 600, 625, 650, 660, 666, 690, 727, 728, 776, 787, 800, 802, 880,1500, 1550, 2008, 2127, 2720, 10000

Secondary: 10, 28, 60, 100, 146, 166, 430, 470, 620, 624, 784, 840, 1600, 1850, 1865, 2050, 2112, 2128, 2213, 2489, 3000, 5000, 5500

Tertiary: 1.2, 7.69, 8, 9.39, 35, 73, 224, 250, 275, 464, 522, 524, 751, 786, 854, 866, 1234, 1800, 2170, 2250, 5148

Suggested points:
DU 4
Jia Ji of UB 23

Yue Ju Wan

Primary: 20, 95, 125, 465, 727, 787, 802, 880, 1550, 5000, 10000

Secondary: 26, 72, 120, 440, 600, 666, 776, 800, 832, 2720, 3000, 6000

Tertiary: 1.1, 1.2, 3, 3.5, 4.9, 7.83, 40, 73, 80, 190, 250, 304, 444, 464, 664, 690, 728, 1552, 1600, 1865, 2008, 2127, 2489

Suggested points:
Jia Ji of UB 18
Jia Ji of UB 20

Yu Nu Jian

Primary: 20, 465, 660, 727, 728, 776, 787, 802, 880, 1550, 1800, 2489, 2720, 10000

Secondary: 95, 120, 166, 428, 430, 440, 444, 464, 470, 600, 620, 624, 625, 650, 690, 784, 800, 832, 840, 1489, 1500, 1600, 1850, 1865, 2008, 2128, 2213, 2950, 3000, 5000

Tertiary: 1.2, 7.69, 10, 28, 35, 46.5, 60, 72, 100, 125, 141, 200, 224, 275, 304, 342, 467, 476, 524, 528, 574, 629, 664, 666, 712, 734, 745, 747, 766, 786, 854, 866, 875, 885, 962, 1000, 1614, 2127, 2170, 5148

Suggested points:
DU 14
Jia Ji of UB 23

Yu Ping Feng San

Primary: 20, 727, 776, 800, 802, 880, 1550, 5000, 10000

Secondary: 120, 125, 146, 428, 440, 444, 465, 522, 660, 676, 688, 728, 760, 766, 786, 832, 1800, 2489, 2720, 3176

Tertiary: 72, 304, 333, 450, 600, 666, 683, 690, 1234, 1488, 1500, 1600, 2008, 2128, 7344

Suggested points:
DU 14
Jia Ji of UB 13

Zhen Gan Xi Feng Tang

Primary: 1.2, 7.83, 10, 20, 72, 95, 125, 465, 470, 600, 650, 727, 787, 800, 802, 880, 1550, 10000

Secondary: 9.6, 26, 60, 120, 166, 430, 444, 620, 624, 625, 660, 690, 728, 776, 840, 1850, 1865, 2008, 2128, 2213, 2720, 3000, 5000, 6000

Tertiary: 1.1, 3.5, 4, 4.9, 5.8, 6, 6.3, 7.69, 9.19, 9.39, 28, 35, 73, 100, 224, 275, 440, 464, 522, 524, 666, 784, 786, 813, 854, 866, 1500, 1600, 1800, 2127, 2170, 2489, 5148

Suggested points:
DU 14
Jia Ji of UB 18

Zhen Wu Tang

Primary: 20, 72, 95, 120, 125, 146, 440, 444, 465, 522, 660, 666, 690, 727, 776, 787, 802, 880, 1550, 5000, 10000

Secondary: 160, 320, 464, 600, 625, 664, 728, 832, 952, 1234, 1500, 1865, 2008, 2050, 2127, 2128, 2250, 2720, 5500

Tertiary: 2, 4.9, 9.39, 10, 40, 73, 100, 190, 424, 650, 682, 741, 800, 987, 1552, 1862, 2112, 2688, 7344

Suggested points:
Jia Ji of UB 20
DU 4

Zhi Bai Di Huang Tang

Primary: 20, 465, 660, 727, 728, 776, 787, 802, 880, 1550, 1800, 2489, 2720, 10000

Secondary: 95, 120, 166, 428, 430, 440, 444, 464, 470, 600, 620, 624, 625, 650, 690, 784, 800, 832, 840, 1489, 1500, 1600, 1850, 1865, 2008, 2128, 2213, 2950, 3000, 5000

Tertiary: 1.2, 7.69, 10, 28, 35, 46.5, 60, 72, 100, 125, 141, 200, 224, 275, 304, 342, 467, 476, 524, 528, 574, 629, 664, 666, 712, 734, 745, 747, 766, 786, 854, 866, 875, 885, 962, 1000, 1614, 2127, 2170, 5148

Suggested points:
DU 14
Jia Ji of UB 23

Zhi Gan Cao Tang

Primary: 10, 20, 40, 72, 95, 120, 125, 428, 440, 444, 464, 465, 620, 625, 650, 660, 666, 676, 690, 727, 728, 760, 776, 784, 786, 787, 800, 802, 880, 1500, 1550, 1600, 1850, 1865, 2008, 2127, 2128, 2489, 2720, 3000, 5000, 10000

Secondary: 1.2, 8, 9.39, 60, 80, 100, 166, 240, 304, 430, 450, 470, 624, 664, 688, 740, 832, 840, 1488, 1800, 1862, 2000, 2112, 2213, 3176

Tertiary: 7.69, 7.83, 28, 35, 47, 73, 160, 220, 224, 250, 275, 400, 422, 424, 500, 524, 622, 712, 727.5, 766, 854, 866, 1234, 1552, 1560, 1570, 2145, 2170, 2250, 3040, 5148, 7344

Suggested points:
Jia Ji of UB 17
Jia Ji of UB 23

Zhi Sou San

Primary: 20, 72, 95, 125, 146, 440, 444, 727, 728, 766, 776, 787, 802, 880, 1234, 1550, 10000

Secondary: 304, 465, 522, 524, 650, 660, 666, 683, 690, 720, 784, 800, 1552, 2008, 2127, 2128, 2182, 2184, 2189, 2217, 2489, 2720, 3176, 3524, 3672, 5000, 7344

Tertiary: 0.5, 7.7, 10, 60, 120, 333, 422, 428, 432, 450, 464, 478, 514, 525, 530, 543, 600, 641, 664, 676, 688, 760, 778, 822, 832, 854, 857, 1050, 1384, 1488, 1500, 1744, 1865, 2000, 2005, 2030, 2048, 2050, 2084, 2100, 2104, 2112, 2116, 2120, 2145, 2160, 2170, 2180, 2876, 2950, 3040, 3702, 3713, 10025, 11780, 17034, 21275

Suggested points:
DU 14
Jia Ji of UB 13

Zhu Ling Tang

Primary: 20, 95, 440, 444, 464, 465, 660, 690, 727, 728, 776, 787, 802, 880, 1500, 1550, 1800, 2128, 2489, 2720, 5000, 10000

Secondary: 72, 120, 125, 146, 160, 166, 320, 428, 430, 470, 522, 600, 620, 624, 625, 650, 666, 766, 784, 800, 832, 840, 952, 1489, 1600, 1850, 1865, 2008, 2050, 2213, 2950, 3000

Tertiary: 1.2, 7.69, 10, 28, 35, 46.5, 60, 100, 141, 200, 224, 275, 304, 342, 467, 476, 524, 528, 574, 629, 664, 682, 712, 734, 741, 745, 747, 786, 854, 866, 875, 885, 962, 987, 1000, 1234, 1614, 1862, 2127, 2170, 2688, 5148

Suggested points:
DU 14
Jia Ji of UB 20

Zhu Ye Shi Gao Tang

Primary: 10, 20, 72, 95, 120, 125, 428, 440, 444, 464, 465, 600, 625, 650, 660, 664, 666, 690, 727, 728, 776, 784, 786, 787, 800, 802, 832, 880, 1500, 1550, 1600, 1800, 1850, 1865, 2008, 2127, 2128, 2489, 2720, 3000, 5000, 10000

Secondary: 1.2, 8, 40, 60, 80, 100, 166, 190, 240, 304, 422, 430, 450, 470, 620, 624, 676, 712, 760, 766, 840, 1000, 1488, 1489, 1552, 2000, 2112, 2213, 2950

Tertiary: 2, 3.9, 4.9, 7.69, 7.83, 9.39, 28, 35, 46.5, 73, 141, 160, 200, 220, 224, 250, 275, 342, 400, 424, 432, 467, 476, 500, 524, 528, 574, 622, 629, 648, 688, 700, 727.5, 732, 734, 740, 745, 747, 854, 866, 875, 885, 962, 1234, 1560, 1570, 1614, 1862, 2170, 2250, 3040, 3176, 5148, 7344

Suggested points:
DU 14
Jia Ji of UB 20

Zou Gui Wan

Primary: 20, 72, 95, 120, 125, 440, 444, 464, 465, 600, 650, 666, 690, 727, 728, 776, 786, 787, 800, 802, 880, 1550, 2008, 2128, 2720, 3000, 5000, 10000

Secondary: 40, 166, 428, 430, 470, 620, 624, 760, 784, 840, 1500, 1600, 1850, 1865, 2127, 2213, 2489

Tertiary: 1.2, 7.69, 10, 28, 35, 60, 100, 146, 224, 250, 275, 524, 676, 688, 854, 866, 1488, 1800, 2000, 2112, 2170, 3176, 5148

Suggested points:
Jia Ji of UB 17
Jia Ji of UB 23

Zuo Jin Wan

Primary: 20, 465, 727, 787, 802, 832, 880, 1550, 10000

Secondary: 26, 476, 660, 747, 776, 800, 1489, 1800, 2489, 2720, 2950

Tertiary: 1.1, 3.5, 7.83, 46.5, 72, 73, 95, 125, 141, 200, 342, 422, 428, 444, 574, 629, 664, 712, 728, 734, 766, 784, 875, 885, 962, 1000, 1500, 1600, 1614, 1865, 6000

Suggested points:
Jia Ji of UB 18
Jia Ji of UB 20

Appendices

BOB BECK PROTOCOLS

Bob Beck was an inventor of alternative health devices, who rediscovered the **Lakhovsky Multiple Wave Oscillator**. He also invented a number of his own devices and developed his own protocols based upon these devices. **Sota Instruments** is the officially endorsed manufacturer of **Bob Beck** devices. **Beck** personally gave them his stamp of approval previously to his death (from a head injury) in 2002.

The Website for **Sota Instruments** is http://www.sota.com

Magnetic Pulser

The **Magnetic Pulser**, or "Magpulser" is a device designed by **Bob Beck** to penetrate deep inside the body to clean out the lymph glands. It is also used for its deeply penetrating effects in cases of chronic herpes or hepatitis infections. Electroherbalism is helpful in dealing with outbreaks, but in cases of chronic, pernicious disease, the magpulser is very useful in deeply penetrating tissue where pathological organisms like to hide. These areas are not always reachable with conventional electroherbalism devices.

The latest **Magnetic Pulser** by **Sota Instruments** is called the MP5. It produces an extremely strong (6,000 Gauss) rapidly pulsed magnetic field. It does not use frequencies.

The device is very easy to use. You simply turn it on, and it will automatically charge and pulse repeatedly for 255 cycles (about 20 minutes,) then it will automatically shut off. You hold the paddle with the magnetic coil close to your body on whatever body part or acupuncture point you wish to expose to the magnetic field. The device does not have to actually be in contact with your body, although the strength of the magnetic field will drop off proportionately with the inverse square law, so it is normal to place the device in contact with the body. Unless you are extremely sensitive, you will not feel anything. It is recommended to use the "negative" side of the magnet, which is clearly marked.

Contra-indications
-Pacemakers: Do not use a magpulser if you have a pacemaker.
-Metallic implants: A magpulser may generate heat or electrical current. Gently test the device first or just don't use it at all.
-Do not place near credit cards, homeopathic remedies or computer discs.

Blood Electrification

The Sota Instruments **Silver Pulser** has a dual function of generating colloidal silver, but also being used as a blood electrification device. To use the Silver Pulser for blood electrification, you attach two electrodes to the skin over the blood vessels in the wrist. The device straps right to the arm. You use it for 2 hours per day, in conjunction with the overall Beck Protocols. The unit will provide a 4 hz AC current.

There is some concern by some people in the alternative health community of transfection, due to electroporation. This occurs when sufficient electricity is introduced to the blood, such that the membranes of the cells will open up and absorb more of whatever substance is in the blood. So for example, if someone was taking medication or drinking alcohol, a smaller amount of this substance would have a much larger effect. However, the **Beck** units do not provide sufficient electricity for this to occur. Still, it is a phenomenon of which to be aware. Care should be taken in initial use of the device, as some people might have heightened sensitivity.

Ozone Water

The Sota Instruments **Water Ozonator** is called the WOZ5. This device functions to ozonate water. This will increase the oxygen content of the water, so that when you drink this water, your body will get extra oxygen.

The device is easy to use. There are 4 time settings, 5 minutes, 15, 30 and 60 minutes. The amount of time you run the device will depend on how much water you would like to ozonate. Larger quantities of water will take a longer time to ozonate. So you adjust the time setting and you connect one end of the hose to the device and put the other end in your water. The hose should produce bubbles in the water. This will tell you that the unit is functioning property.

One should use a glass container for the water, as the ozone might react with plastic.

If you have sensitivity, or a preference against the fragrance produced by ozone, run the device on a stove with a ventilator above it. Alternatively, you could open a window or provide some other sort of ventilation.

Drink the water while it is fresh, as the ozone water has a very short half life. The ozone will also function to kill germs in the water.

Colloidal Silver

There is a great deal of confusion, hysteria and misinformation about colloidal silver. Our aim here is to provide an authoritative source for reference. However, do not take the information we provide here as the last word. Research is ongoing, and more information may arise. Our information derives from Dr. Mercola's popular web site and from www.silversafety.org

The classical colloidal silver discussion forum is at http://silverlist.org/

There are mimimal risks to excessive silver intake. The main risk is that of argyria, which is the bluish/greyish coloring of the skin. To avoid this, use the "Silver Safety Calculation."

The formula for this is 12x(body height)/ppm=number of drops per day. PPM means "parts per million," which is a measure of the strength of the silver colloid solution. The number of drops for short term use (about 10 days per month) would be about 120x(body weight)/ppm=number of drops per day. 306,600x(body weight)/ppm=number of drops for your entire lifetime.

This will prevent your intake of silver from becoming more than 25% of your daily allowable intake, according to the EPA.

When you use a generator to make your own colloidal silver, use distilled water. Distilled water has all the minerals and impurities removed. A water filter will not suffice for this purpose. Do not add salt to the water.

There are three main types of "colloidal silver."

One type is "**ionic silver.**" Ionic particles are smaller than regular colloidal silver, so they have a smaller surface area. There is less silver in the solution for the same amount of water as regular colloidal silver. It is effective, but not as much as colloidal silver. It has a low risk of argyria.

A second type of colloidal silver is **silver protein**. These particles are larger than regular colloidal silver, and they are bound together with protein. However these silver particles actually have less surface area than the other forms of silver. The risk of argyria with silver protein is considered to be high, because of the large concentration of silver particles. Silver protein will generally have a very high ppm.

The third type of colloidal silver is "true" **colloidal silver**. According to Mercola, true colloidal silver will not cause argyria, because of the small particle size and the low concentration of ionic particles.

Silver Pulser

The **Silver Pulser** is Sota's colloidal silver generator. It is designed according to **Beck's** specifications, and it can also be used for blood electrification. To make colloidal silver, put the silver electrodes into a container of water and turn the power on for the specified amount of time. Use only distilled water. The silver will react chemically to impurities in the water.

Studies

Current Science, Vol. 91, No. 7, October 10, 2006, Department of Microbiology/Molecular Biology of Brigham-Young University,
"Silver–Water–DispersionTM solution has been shown as an effective antibiotic against many Methicillin-resistant Staphylococcus aureus (MRSA) and multiple drug-resistant (MDR) strains (Escherichia coli, Pseudomonas aeruginosa)."

Nanomedicine: Nonotechnology, Biology and Medicine Vol. 3, Issue 2, June 2007, Pages 168–171Department of Pharmaceutical Biotechnology and Medical Nanotechnology Research Center, Faculty of Pharmacy and Medical Sciences at the University of Tehran, Iran.
"The antibacterial activities of penicillin G, amoxicillin, erythromycin, clindamycin, and vancomycin were increased in the presence of Ag-NPs against both test strains."

Colloids Surface B Interfaces 2007 Oct 1;59(2):171-8. Epub 2007 May 18. Formation of colloidal silver nanoparticles stabilized by Na+-poly(gamma-glutamic acid)-silver nitrate complex via chemical reduction process. Department of Textile Science, Nanya Institute of Technology, Chung-Li, Tao-Yuan, Taiwan.

Journal of Physical Chemistry B, 2006 Aug 24;110(33):16248-53. Department of Physical Chemistry, Palacký University, Svobody 26, 771 46 Olomouc, Czech Republic.
"...silver particles with a narrow size distribution with an average size of 25 nm, which showed high antimicrobial and bactericidal activity against Gram-positive and Gram-negative bacteria, including highly multi-resistant strains such as methicillin-resistant Staphylococcus aureus (MRSA). The study further demonstrated that very low concentrations of silver could be utilized to destroy MRSA, as long as the silver particles were very small, averaging 25 nm."

Chelation Protocols

The following are protocols for argyria. This will help chelate silver out of the body in cases of excess silver accumulation. They are taken from **Nenah Sylver's** excellent **Handbook of Rife Frequency Therapy,** page 263.

Every morning with one quart of water:

-200 mcg of yeast-free selenium (safe to take on an ongoing basis)

-Vitamin E, 100% mixed with tocopherols (d-alpha, beta, delta and gamma tocopherols.) People over 50 who may be at risk for stroke should take 1000 IU. Those under 50 who are not at risk of stroke should take 2000 IU per day. Since high doses of Vitamin E thins the blood, check with your doctor. This supplement may be contraindicated for people on medication to thicken the blood, hemophiliacs and other high risk individuals.

-2 teaspoons of organic MSM (Sulphur, or MSM, also binds with silver and helps pull it from the body.)

-4,000 mg (4 grams) of Vitamin C per day, in 1000-mg (1-gram) doses each.

-1 high potency Vitamin B-complex tablet, 100 mg

-1 teaspoon kelp powder. (You might be able to substitute ¼ -1 teaspoon of liquid colloidal iodine.)

-Liquid or ionic minerals, including trace minerals, 2 ounces or more a day. Minerals containing fulvic acid work better than a formula without fulvic acid.

In addition to the water you take with the above supplements, drink another ¾ of a gallon (6 quarts or 6 liters) of water a day.

-Adapted from www.silvermedicine.com/forumviewtopic.php?t=13 and www.silverproducts.com/argyria.html

HULDA CLARK

Hulda Clark was a Naturopath who believed that diseases generally stem from parasitic infections. This may seem a bit odd to many people, but recall that, according to the pleomorphic theory, these parasites might be considered to be part of the normal life cycle of pathogens in a diseased body. In this case, the main pathogenic factor would be toxic exposure, resulting from diet, environment or other lifestyle factors. Also consider that, strictly speaking, bacteria and viruses are parasitical.

Hulda Clark's unconventional views caused her to have problems practicing her medical theories in the US, so for many years she practiced at **Century Nutrition Clinic** in Tijuana, Mexico. Her books contain a copyright release for reproduction of the intellectual content, and the schematics for her electro-medicine devices are given out for free. She passed away in 2009, due to complications resulting from a car accident.

Zapper

The **Zapper** is very similar to an electroherbalism machine. The main difference is that it has a much smaller frequency range. As a result it is considerably less expensive. The device is usually used with hand tubes, although it can be adapted for foot plates as well. We would probably alter it for electro-acupuncture or use TENS pads to apply the impulse to specific acupuncture points, like Ren 12 or ST 25.

These units are made to kill parasites, especially Candida Albicans.

Clark normally recommended zapping once a day for at least a month, then dropping down to twice a week afterwards. One session will usually take about an hour, although many people will just zap until they subjectively begin to feel better. It is also recommended to drink plenty of water, to prepare the body for a Herxheimer reaction.

Syncrometer

The **Syncrometer** is a diagnostic device. It will match the frequency of a substance you put on the sensor plate to frequencies inside your body. It can scan the body for objects. You put saliva or a body part on one plate, and a sample of a pathogen on the other plate. You also hold a copper hand tube. The device will give you a number of different sounds, based upon positive, negative or neutral detection results.

Green Black Walnut Tincture

Clark also recommended **Green Black Walnut Tincture** as an anti-parasitic treatment. This is Black Walnut, tinctured while still green. This is not an electro-medicine device, but we thought we would simply mention it here in the interest of being veracious.

MICRO-ELECTRICITY GERM KILLER

The **Micro Electricity Germ Killer** comes in two different types. These are the **Godzilla** and the **GodRod**. They both use low voltage direct current and function to electrocute germs. You make them yourself with batteries, so they are very inexpensive.

Direct current is different from alternating current, in that it does not have a frequency. In alternating current, the signal reverses direction every so often. This directional reversal is its frequency. However direct current continues to flow only in one direction. Therefore these devices do not function based on the principle of resonant frequencies, or "Mortal Oscillatory Rates," but on straight up electrocution of the pathogenic microbes.

http://health.groups.yahoo.com/group/microelectricitygermkiller/

and

http://health.groups.yahoo.com/group/microelectricitygermkiller2/

are forums where these devices are discussed. They have many files of testimonials and independent studies created by individual researchers who casually participated in the groups. It should be noted however, that these groups are not peer reviewed. These people are not credentialed scientists, and as such are not recognized as a "panel of knowledgeable experts" by the mainstream establishment.

We do not have much experience with these devices, but we have decided to include them and allow you all to experiment with them and decide for yourselves. Electricity is considered to be a "flow of electrons," where electrons are sub-atomic particles. We can consider them to be "quanta" of qi. Therefore we can hypothesize that in applying these devices to specific points, we may be "tonifying qi" on those points.

Godzilla

As always, we are self published authors, so in the interest of keeping the price of our books down, we avoid including diagrams, photographs or illustrations of any type. We want to keep them affordable for you. However, at the links provided above you will find schematics and photos that will assist you in the construction of a **Godzilla** device.

These low cost devices are easy to construct. You simply take a square 9 volt battery and attach wires to the two connectors at the top of the battery. You run these wires to sponges. The sponges should be natural sponges. You can also use pieces of cloth. The main thing you want is that, the sponge or cloth should be able to retain water. This water will conduct the electrical current.

Now you wet the sponges and apply them to the body. Let's say you have an infection in your hand. You would put one of the sponges, which is functioning as an electrode on the palmar side of your hand and one on the back of your hand. This will create a circuit through which electricity will flow from one of the connectors on the battery to the other. The electricity, while flowing through your hand will (it is claimed) kill the infection.

These devices (it is claimed) are great for dental infections. For that purpose you would obviously use something smaller than a sponge, as you would put the electrodes on the gums on either side of the tooth. You could also likely place them on opposite sides of your face. Check the yahoogroups listed above for discussions of how other people have done it, and what has worked and not worked for them.

They are also recommended for treating pain.

It is usually recommended to switch the electrodes around every 5 minutes or so.

Godrods

Godrods are the same thing as a **Godzilla**, but they use C or D cell batteries, in line with each other. So they are **Godzillas**, but in the form of a rod. Hence, **Godrod**. You tape or fasten the two batteries together, so that the bottom of one is connected to the top of the other. Then you use a sponge on the bottom of the series of batteries and the top of the series of batteries.

As you press down with one hand on the bottom sponge, you will press the batteries and the top sponge onto the site of the infection. In our case, we might consider putting this onto an acupuncture point. But this pressing of the batteries with wet sponges will create a circuit for the direct current, through the top of the battery, into the site of the infection (or acupuncture point) then down to the hand and up into the bottom of the other battery through the wet sponge on the bottom of the **Godrod**. There are photos at the above yahoogroups which make things much clearer.

It's the same device as the **Godzilla**, but it uses different types of batteries.

SCENAR

The **Scenar** is a Russian device. It was developed for their space program. Their cosmonauts are not trained in medicine, per se, and as they recycle urine for water on board the space station, they did not want the cosmonauts to be using drugs.

Scenar (with a hard "k" sound) stands for **Self-Controlled Energo Neuro Adaptive Regulation**. There are many makes and models of these devices. There is also a professional grade version and a "home use" version, which is less fancy but also less expensive. They function to stimulate biofeedback to promote healing.

There are two ways to use a scenar. The first is to simply rub the device in an x pattern along the problem area to be treated. If the device gets stuck, or is harder to push along the surface of the skin in one direction moreso than the other, then you continue rubbing the device in that direction, either vertically or horizontally across the body. Do this until the resistance fades.

Note that the power on the device should be turned on, and it should be set to a high enough level of power so that the person can comfortably tolerate the stimulation. This will mean that, it will not be turned up as high on the head. But if you wanted to use it on a person's back or chest, you could reasonably turn the power up higher.

This is said to stimulate a healing response from the brain, to increase the regeneration of the problem area. We suspect that, like the Micro Electricity Germ Killer, what the scenar is doing is tonifying qi to the area, and also is very likely promoting the movement of qi and blood.

The device will treat pain, but it will also (or is said to) promote healing.

The second way to use the device is to put it on an acupuncture or trigger point. The device will then apply a flow of direct current to that point, and will automatically shut off when it senses that the point does not require further treatment. There are separate settings for each of these functions.

MRSA

MRSA is an anti-biotic resistant form of Staph Aureus bacteria. This is one type of infection that can be very difficult to treat with conventional means. We have had some anecdotal success treating this condition. These are our methods.

Method 1: Electro-Acupuncture

We will usually use TENS pads on **MRSA**. You can run the electricity through needles, but the TENS pads have a larger surface area, hence will give a stronger connection.

The frequencies, as always, are derived from this list:
http://www.electroherbalism.com/Bioelectronics/FrequenciesandAnecdotes/CAFL.htm
Staph infection_1 - 943, 727, 643, 20
Staph_and_Strep_v - 40887, 9646, 7160, 2431, 1902, 1109, 1060, 1050, 1010, 985, 958, 934, 786, 727, 718, 686, 643, 576, 563, 542, 453, 436, 423, 411, 333, 134, 128
Staphylococci_infection (see also other Staph freqs, 727*, 786*) - 960, 727, 786, 453, 678, 674, 550, 1109, 424, 943, 1050, 643, 2600, 7160, 639, 1089, 8697
Staphylococcus_aureus (can cause boils, carbuncles, abscesses, tooth infection, heart disease, and infect tumors, 786*) - 8697, 7270, 1050, 999, 943, 824.4, 787, 784, 745, 738, 728, 727, 647, 644, 555, 478, 424
Staphylococcus_aureus_HC (tooth infection, abscesses, heart disease, invades tumors) - 18819.51, 936.97, 18968.87, 944.40
Staphylococcus_comp - 40887, 9646, 8697, 7270, 7160, 2600, 2431, 1902, 1109, 1089, 1060, 1050, 1010, 999, 985, 960, 958, 943, 934, 884, 882, 880, 878, 876, 824.4, 787, 786, 784, 745, 738, 728, 727, 718, 686, 678, 674, 647, 644, 643, 639, 634, 576, 563, 555, 550, 542, 478, 453, 436, 424, 423, 411, 333, 134, 128
Staphylococcus_general (728*, 786*) - 7160, 1109, 1089, 885, 884, 883, 882, 881, 880, 879, 878, 877, 876, 875, 786, 728, 674, 639, 634, 550, 453

CAUTIONS:
-Do not use this method if the person has electrical issues with their heart.
-Do not use on pregnant women or epileptics. Or small children.
-Do not use on transplantees.
-Do at least three treatments, to make sure that you kill all of the bacteria.
-Allow 2-3 days for the body to rid itself of die-off. Drink plenty of water.
-Use caution in case of metallic implants.

Method 2: Essential Oils

We've already written a book on this, although we did not create a specific section for killing MRSA. We might go back and add that.

Cinnamon oil is the best. I will usually prefer Cinnamon Bark, but according to these studies, Cinnamon Leaf works great too. Eucalyptus, Tea tree, Thyme white, Lavender, Lemon, Lemongrass, Grapefruit, Clove Bud, Sandalwood, Peppermint, Kunzea and Sage are all covered and vouched for. Be careful with Cinnamon, as it can burn.

http://www.ncbi.nlm.nih.gov/pubmed/19473851
J Craniomaxillofac Surg. 2009 Oct;37(7):392-7. doi: 10.1016/j.jcms.2009.03.017. Epub 2009 May 26.
The battle against multi-resistant strains: Renaissance of antimicrobial essential oils as a promising force to fight hospital-acquired infections.
Warnke PH, Becker ST, Podschun R, Sivananthan S, Springer IN, Russo PA, Wiltfang J, Fickenscher H, Sherry E.
Department of Oral and Maxillofacial Surgery, University of Kiel, Germany. warnke@mkg.uni-kiel.de
"Several common and hospital-acquired bacterial and yeast isolates (6 Staphylococcus strains including MRSA, 4 Streptococcus strains and 3 Candida strains including Candida krusei) were tested for their susceptibility for Eucalyptus, Tea tree, Thyme white, Lavender, Lemon, Lemongrass, Cinnamon, Grapefruit, Clove Bud, Sandalwood, Peppermint, Kunzea and Sage oil with the agar diffusion test. Olive oil, Paraffin oil, Ethanol (70%), Povidone iodine, Chlorhexidine and hydrogen peroxide (H(2)O(2)) served as controls. Large prevailing effective zones of inhibition were observed for Thyme white, Lemon, Lemongrass and Cinnamon oil. The other oils also showed considerable efficacy. Remarkably, almost all tested oils demonstrated efficacy against hospital-acquired isolates and reference strains, whereas Olive and Paraffin oil from the control group produced no inhibition. As proven in vitro, essential oils represent a cheap and effective antiseptic topical treatment option even for antibiotic-resistant strains as MRSA and antimycotic-resistant Candida species."

http://www.ncbi.nlm.nih.gov/pubmed/11483389
J Ethnopharmacol. 2001 Sep;77(1):123-7.
Antibacterial activity of leaf essential oils and their constituents from Cinnamomum osmophloeum.
Chang ST, Chen PF, Chang SC.
Department of Forestry, National Taiwan University, No 1 Section 4, Roosevelt, Taipei, Taiwan, ROC.
peter@ms.cc.ntu.edu.tw

"The nine strains of bacteria, including Escherichia coli, Pseudomonas aeruginosa, Enterococcus faecalis, Staphylococcus aureus, Staphylococcus epidermidis, methicillin-resistant Staphylococcus aureus (MRSA), Klebsiella pneumoniae, Salmonella sp., and Vibrio parahemolyticus, were used in the antibacterial tests. Results from the antibacterial tests demonstrated that the indigenous cinnamon B leaf essential oils had an excellent inhibitory effect. The MICs (minimum inhibitory concentrations) of the B leaf oil were 500 microg/ml against both K. pneumoniae and Salmonella sp. and 250 microg/ml against the other seven strains of bacteria. Cinnamaldehyde possessed the strongest antibacterial activity compared to the other constituents of the essential oils. The MICs of cinnamaldehyde against the E. coli, P. aeruginosa, E. faecalis, S. aureus, S. epidermidis, MRSA, K. pneumoniae, Salmonella sp., and V. parahemolyticus were 500, 1000, 250, 250, 250, 250, 1000, 500, and 250 microg/ml, respectively. These results suggest that C. osmophloeum leaf essential oil and cinnamaldehyde are beneficial to human health, having the potential to be used for medical purposes and to be utilized as anti-bacterial additives in making paper products. "

http://www.ncbi.nlm.nih.gov/pubmed/21941919
Nat Prod Commun. 2011 Sep;6(9):1379-84.
Role of direct bioautographic method for detection of antistaphylococcal activity of essential oils.
Horváth G, Jámbor N, Kocsis E, Böszörményi A, Lemberkovics E, Héthelyi E, Kovács K, Kocsis B.Institute of Pharmacognosy, Medical School, University of Pécs, Pécs, Hungary. gyorgyi.horvath@aok.pte.hu
"The aim of the present study was the chemical characterization of some traditionally used and therapeutically relevant essential oils (thyme, eucalyptus, cinnamon bark, clove, and tea tree) and the optimized microbiological investigation of the effect of these oils on clinical isolates of methicillin-resistant Staphylococcus aureus (MRSA) and methicillin-susceptible S. aureus (MSSA). The chemical composition of the oils was analyzed by TLC, and controlled by gas chromatography (GC) and gas chromatography/mass spectrometry (GC/MS). The antibacterial effect was investigated using a TLC-bioautographic method. Antibacterial activity of thyme, clove and cinnamon oils, as well as their main components (thymol, carvacrol, eugenol, and cinnamic aldehyde) was observed against all the bacterial strains used in this study. The essential oils of eucalyptus and tea tree showed weak activity in the bioautographic system. "

http://onlinelibrary.wiley.com/doi/10.1111/j.1472-765X.2008.02406.x/abstract
Comparison of bacteriostatic and bactericidal activity of 13 essential oils against strains with varying sensitivity to antibiotics
1. L. Mayaud1, A. Carricajo2, A. Zhiri3, G. Aubert1
Article first published online: 22 AUG 2008
Letters in Applied Microbiology

"Conclusions: Cinnamomum verum bark had the highest antimicrobial activity, particularly against resistant strains. Significance and Impact of the Study: Bacteriostatic and bactericidal activity of EO on nosocomial antibiotic-resistant strains. "

CAUTIONS:
-Do not use on pregnant women or epileptics, (without permission from an MD.)
-Some oils can be photosensitive.
-Menthol oils should not be used on children under 3.
-Do not apply to inner ear.
-Dilute if used on the head. We will dilute them with a carrier anyway, there's a section on this in our book.
-Keep away from eyes. If oils are on your finger, don't scratch your eyes.
-Test the oil for sensitivity. People can have reactions.
-Keep oils away from fire.
-Avoid mucous membranes.
-Some oils have an estrogenic property.
-Drink plenty of water. Detoxification may occur.
SEE: Essential Oil Safety by Tisserand.

Method 3: Colloidal Silver

We covered **colloidal silver** in the section under **Bob Beck** Protocols.

The problem with CS is that it will kill the **MRSA**, but the **MRSA** will come back. It will usually come back 2-3 times, weaker each time. But then it will go away. See section on **Bob Beck** Protocols.

CAUTIONS:
-Use distilled water if you make it yourself. Do not add salt or other compounds.
-Avoid silver protein
-Don't overdose.

Method 4: Allicin C

This product is a garlic extract. We've never tried it, but according to their advertisements, they test every batch against **MRSA** to make sure it's strong enough. Regular garlic won't touch **MRSA**.

Method 5: Godzilla

The **Godzilla** is a simple low voltage direct current. Run some speaker wires off of a 9 volt battery, into two wetted sponges. Apply locally to the infected area. See section on **Godzilla**.

HARMONICS

When we speak of harmonics, there are two things we might mean. There are **wave harmonics** and there are **function harmonics**. Both are an important part of electroherbalism.

Wave Harmonics

Sometimes a frequency generator will have a limited range of frequencies. For example, one Lyme's Disease frequency is 27,735,768. Many frequency generators will not go that high. So what you do is you generate a wave half that size.

Imagine a wave that is 10 feet long. Now imagine a wave that is 5 feet long. The 5 foot wave will complete itself halfway through that 10 foot wave, but then the second 5 foot long wave will hit that same frequency as the 10 foot wave. So if you can't generate a 10 foot wave, you can generate a 5 foot wave. Now many people will also say to run this shorter wave for twice as long. Experiment, see what works for you. But a 5 foot wave should harmonize with that 10 foot wave.

The square wave will, by its structure create more harmonics than other wave forms, such as sine waves.

Function Harmonics

Function harmonics are what allow us to create frequency lists based upon the traditional herbal formulas. A function harmonic is a frequency that performs two or more functions, which are needed in a given treatment.

Let's say we want to nourish yin and move qi and blood. We would look at the frequency lists and find numbers that are included in both. Then we would run those numbers to perform both functions simultaneously. This allows us to perform an easy and efficient treatment for both conditions simultaneously, especially when combined with the correct points. In some cases, several function harmonics are required.

NOVOBIOTRONICS

http://novobiotronics.com/

NovoBioTronics is a 501(c)(3) nonprofit scientific research & educational organization dedicated to discovering and developing new approaches and techniques in the use of electronic technology for biological and biomedical research. NovoBioTronics actively explores areas where modern electronic technologies can help form a synergistic nexus with biological and biomedical research. We engage in laboratory experimentation as well as research and development of state of the art customized electronic technologies which may have biological and biomedical applications. Novobiotronics has made major advances in the use of a noninvasive and nontoxic electronic treatment of human cancer cells and antibiotic resistant bacteria.

Novobiotronics, Inc.
PO Box 1210
Sarasota Springs NY, 12866
Info@Novobiotronics.com

Donate:
http://www.novobiotronics.com/Donate.html

BIBLIOGRAPHY

Becker, Robert, **The Body Electric: Electromagnetism And The Foundation Of Life**

Clark, Hulda, **The Cure for all Diseases**

Clement, Mark, **The Waves that Heal**

Enby, Gosch, Sheehan, **Hidden Killers: The Revolutionary Discoveries of Gunther Enderlein**

Enderlein, Gunther, **Life Cycle of Bacteria**

Hume, David, **Enquiry Concerning Human Understanding**

Lakhovsky, George, **The Secret of Life**

Lynes, Barry, **Rife's World of Electromedicine**

McInturff, Brian, **The Electroherbalism Frequency Lists**

Peirce, Charles Sanders, **Philosophical Writings**

Popper, Karl R, **The Logic of Scientific Discovery**

Rosner, Bryan, et al. **When Antibiotics Fail: Lyme Disease and Rife Machines, with Critical Evaluation of Leading Alternative Therapies**

Sylver, Nenah, **The Rife Handbook of Frequency Therapy and Holistic Health**

Tisserand, **Essential Oil Safety**

Whitehead, Alfred North, **Process and Reality**

Whitehead, Alfred North, **Science and the Modern World**

FURTHER WEB SITES

http://www.nenahsylver.com/

http://www.kentbergstrom.com

http://www.bubishi.com

http://www.mercola.com

http://www.electroherbalism.com/

http://health.groups.yahoo.com/group/Beck-blood-electrification/

http://health.groups.yahoo.com/group/Beck-n-stuff/

http://health.groups.yahoo.com/group/DrClark/

http://health.groups.yahoo.com/group/drloyd/

http://health.groups.yahoo.com/group/electroherbalism/

http://health.groups.yahoo.com/group/microelectricitygermkiller/

http://health.groups.yahoo.com/group/microelectricitygermkiller2/